The Living End

A wellness guide to the dying process

by

Judith P. Hereford RN MSN

Copyright © 1983, 1992, 2019 by Judith Hereford
All rights reserved. This book or any portion thereof
may not be reproduced or used in any manner whatsoever
without the express written permission of the publisher
except for the use of brief quotations in a book review.
Printed in the United States of America

Second edition, 2019

ISBN 1087079769

RLC Publication
6400 Minnesota Ave
Saint Louis, MO 63111

www.ahereford.org

Table of Contents

INTRODUCTION..1

1. THE WELLNESS OF DYING......................................5

2. SPIRITUAL WELLNESS..15

3. MENTAL WELLNESS...23

4. EMOTIONAL WELLNESS...29

5. PHYSICAL WELLNESS...39
    THE CIRCULATORY SYSTEM..40
    THE KIDNEYS...57
    THE RESPIRATORY SYSTEM..65
    THE NERVOUS SYSTEM..79
    THE DIGESTIVE SYSTEM..95

SOME FINAL COMMENTS...107

REFERENCES..113

GLOSSARY...115

List of Figures

Figure 1: The Human Heart..44

Figure 2: Cardiac Cycle...45

Figure 3: Circulatory System......................................47
Figure 4: The Kidneys...58
Figure 5: The Kidney Interior....................................59
Figure 6: The Lungs..67
Figure 7: Chest Cavity..68
Figure 8: The Chest with Lungs Visible....................69
Figure 9: The brain Inside the Scull..........................80
Figure 10: The Nervous System................................81
Figure 11: The Brain..83
Figure 12: Brain with Spinal Cord.............................84
Figure 13: Abdominal Digestive Organs...................97
Figure 14: The Digestive System..............................99

Introduction

Any time you are at a meeting or party or gathering of people, and you want some privacy, just say this, "Let's all talk about our own impending death." I guarantee that in short order you will have an abundance of elbow room. The fact is most people don't like to talk or even think about dying. In modern American culture our values are centered around youth and vitality. Television, movies, and music all focus on the here and now, and on every aspect of being alive-- beauty, relationships, money, ambition, success. All this media input distracts us from the inevitable progression of time, and the progression of life into death. Through all our efforts to battle wrinkles and gray hair and sagging thighs, we have managed to convince ourselves that somehow, some way, we don't have to die. If we just don't think about it, it won't happen to us. But the truth is, it will happen to us, and to people that we love; and while it is not healthy to constantly dwell on the topic and become morbid about it, it is very important to be informed. Perhaps no one can truly be prepared for death; however knowledge about the precedes that proceeds it can remove some of our fears about death and put us more at ease in approaching it ourselves, or with someone we love.

One reason many of us are so afraid to contemplate death is that it is an unfamiliar experience. With a few rare exceptions each of us only gets one shot at it. We don't get the chance to get comfortable, to get good at it. With most new things in our lives we are nervous the first time we do them, and as they become familiar, we become more secure. For example, your second week at a new job, you are able to visualize where you will park your car, the people you will interact with, the places you will be spending time, etc. With these mental images, you are able to prepare yourself for the coming day.

But this is not the case when you think about an approaching death. Most of us don't know what will happen to us, how we will feel, or what changes will take place in our bodies. We have systematically detached ourselves from death with hospitals and nursing homes. These institutions may seem to shield us from death, but in fact the shroud of mystery they create only enhances our fears. Even if someone close to you has died, unless you were near during the final days and weeks of life, and understood the progression that was taking place, death can still be an incomprehensible event.

You may argue that it is impossible to understand death-- that people have unsuccessfully sought these answers for centuries. I don't pretend to have discovered the philosophical or theological secrets of dying. However, there are certain normal physical events that occur when the body is dying, and this is the mystery that I hope to illuminate in this book. For non-medical people, and even medical professionals, these chapters are a practical guide to the dying process. I will explain the changes that come about in the body as death nears, why these things are taking place, what action should be taken, and more importantly, what action should not be taken.

Aside from removing some of the anxiety associated with dying, this information will help you to remain in control of the situation as death nears. Although medical professionals have the best of intentions, it is the dying person and their loved ones who should be making decisions. Should the dying person be at home or in the hospital? Should medical treatment continue or should nature be allowed to run its course? What physical events should be fought and what should merely be noted as a normal part of a natural process? With the knowledge contained in this book, you will be better informed to make these decisions and many others that you will face.

The Living End

1. The Wellness of Dying

Given the choice we would all select to be fully WELL. We do not like to think about having any type of malfunction with which to deal. We want perfect health, perfect relationships, perfect careers, perfect families, and perfect emotions. This is what makes disease, illness and dying so difficult for us. Donald Ardell, who many believe is the father of the modern wellness movement, says that it is possible to be "well" even amid disease and dying. He continues:

> "You can learn to accept the eventuality of your own mortality - and experience the dying process as another aspect of human reality. If ì you do this, neither illness nor the acceptance of eventual death will inhibit your acceptance of life - and the treasuring of optimal ì good health

> that will enable you to achieve the fullest existence within your potential. For there is always illness and death in wellness and life and, in the last analysis, the ratio between birth and death will be one-to-one."

In the dying process we are dealing with a body that is deteriorating, but the rest of the person can be well. In our society when a person becomes diseased they become consumed by the condition and allow the whole of the person to be ill. In disease or injury we tend to focus so completely on the body and it's imperfections that we lose ourselves and then become totally not well.

Health includes all the dimensions of life working in harmony to produce a sense of well-being and peace. The dimensions of life include not only the physical, but the emotions, the mind and the spirit. It takes into account our relationships, our need for learning, our hopes and dreams and our need for God.

In the wellness movement we know that we need balance among the physical, mental, spiritual, and emotional aspects of our life. We need to develop all parts of us to be really whole. This is to our advantage because when we have one part stressed the other elements can fill in to keep us going.

We are aware of what makes us physically well. It is when all our body parts are working well enough so that we don't have to pay a lot of attention to them. When we have a headache we, suddenly become very mindful of that big round ball sitting on top of our shoulders pounding away. It is not until someone asked about that headache that we suddenly remember the ache as well as the head. Today's society encourages us to be physically fit. Often this is what people call wellness. This is just one aspect of the whole picture.

You are spiritually well when you have good relationships with many beings. You need to get your needs met by association with others. We in the wellness movement believe that it is necessary to have a relationship with a supreme being. You all need time to be alone and to just "be". It is also essential to have someone with whom to share yourself. You need someone who can challenge you, someone to support you emotionally, someone to tell you when you are wrong or unreasonable. These are some of the essentials for spiritual wellness.

One of the most important aspects of emotional wellness is liking yourself. Each of us is a unique individual and each one of us has things that are likable. We need to know who we are before we can like ourselves. Most of us were educated to always think of the other fellow. We were told in childhood that it was selfish to always think of our own needs. This is true, but unfortunately we carried that into adulthood believing that we should never think about ourselves. "Love thy neighbor as thy self." You can't love anyone if you don't love yourself first.

Mental wellness is not just the absence of psychosis. Mental wellness is being alert and eager to learn new things. It is being aware of your internal and external surroundings. Mentally well people don't need to be sick to take a day off to do just what they want to do.

It is taking control of yourself and working with the body to stay as well as possible. It is using the immune system to ward off infection and other foreign invaders.

We know that the stresses of life can challenge any part of us. Our wellness attitude can keep us in balance and get us through. When you are exposed to the common cold you probably tell yourself that you will "get a cold". Sure enough several days later the symptoms appear. You have given yourself permission to suffer that cold. However, have you ever been around a cold epidemic, but told yourself you were too busy for a cold right now? Then later you were amazed to realize that you were one of the few people who didn't suffer from that round of colds. Was this coincidence? No. When you told yourself that you didn't have time for the cold, you also alerted your immune system to get busy and do what your body does best. Take care of you.

You reach wellness by giving some time and attention to "ALL" of you everyday, or at least an average of that. There are people who don't take days off and never take a vacation. There are those who meditate each day, but never exercise. Some of us sit up all night reading and start the new day with less than adequate sleep. We all need rest, relaxation, exercise, balanced nutrition, intellectual stimulation, meditation and conversation -- all this is necessary for WELLNESS.

When one dimension of a person is met with difficulty "wellness people" call on the unhindered aspects to see them through the difficult time. You break your leg.

The Living End

A cast is applied and you have difficulty getting around. You are no longer physically well. You are, however, still well spiritually, emotionally, and mentally, given that these were in balance before the fracture occurred. In the wellness lifestyle you will use these other aspects to get you through the broken leg.

Using your spiritual wellness you will rely on your friends and family to help you get around, because you have a relationship with them that allows you to feel comfortable accepting their help. They will also cheer you up and entertain you with cards and flowers. Your mental wellness will allow you to encourage your bone to heal and use the down time that you have to catch up on your reading. You will be free to read the novels that you have on your "I want to read" list.

Emotional wellness allows you to see the good that can come from this accident. You will not be chastising yourself for the accident, but realize that no one is perfect and that it is okay for you to have an accident. So, you see, a wellness attitude can help you stay balanced through all the pleasant or disagreeable events in your life.

How does this wellness concept apply to the dying process? Life is a continuum. The journey begins at birth and ends at death. All along the journey we can chose to be well and whole accentuating the positive or we can worry about all that we do not have and concentrate on the negative.

When you were born your body was at the peak of its youth and vitality, but your mental, emotional and spiritual powers were almost non- existent. As you grew and developed the high peak in the physical diminished as the other aspects began to develop. As an adult who practices wellness techniques these will be in balance throughout the most of your life.

During the dying process the body loses physical wellness. We know that this will be a permanent loss, unlike the lack of physical wellness with the broken leg. During this time there is no reason the mental, emotional and spiritual aspects of the person cannot compensate for this decrease in the physical. The problem in today's society is that when the body becomes less than perfect the whole person takes on the "sick role." It is your choice, YOU can be well even when your body is less than perfect.

You learn the rewards of the "sick role" very young. When you don't feel well you get much attention. You don't have to go to school, you get presents, you don't have to do your chores. You get to watch television and someone fixes special food for you. When you grow up you are entitled to "sick days" not "well days." Our society rewards "being sick"; it does not reward "being well."

We also learn about dying. The adults talk about someone who is very ill in hushed tones and they have sad expressions on their faces. Children are told to be solemn and silent around the dying. Nothing is explained about what is happening. You only hear words like: tragic, terrible, awful, dreadful, shocking, appalling. You, as a child, begin to associate these words with the dying process and you learn to fear dying. There is a great song from South Pacific which explains that "you have to be taught to hate and fear.

The Living End

You have to be taught year after year." So we learn to fear dying and we carry that fear into our adult life.

As you grow you have other experiences with death that shape your attitude. When your kitten or puppy died you were sad. You felt a lose and your parents helped you have a funeral for the pet to help you through this separation time.

When your grandparent, aunt or uncle died you watched your parents as they grieved and you saw how your first teachers handled the loss of a loved one. If the person who died endured a lingering illness, you were exposed to the dying process. You witnessed the work, pain, difficulty, and frightening events that sometimes accompany dying when the participants are ignorant about the natural process.

You have watched many dying scenes in the movies and on television. We are all influenced by the way death is presented in the media. Movies like Gone With the Wind, Brian's Song, Arthur, Amadeus, and Bang the Drums Slowly portray someone who is dying. We must remember that while the dying scene is based on real experiences it is depicted from the director's perspective. Such films are not aimed at educating us about dying. They are telling a story and the purpose of the dying scenes is to move the story line along.

Literature is full of an author's view of dying. Many times an author will attempt to put the reader inside the skin of the dying person to make them experience what that character is feeling. Again, it is that author's own interpretation of what dying is about based on personal experience.

We know that movies and novels are make believe, but this exposure to the dying of others does have an impact on our feelings about death. We tuck these emotions away in our subconscious mind without really processing it for our own use. We reason that death occurs to other people and doesn't affect us. We will worry about it later.

The day finally does come when we are face to face with dying. Either you are diagnosed with a progressive illness or someone in your inner circle receives such a pronouncement. Suddenly death is not something that happens to others. It is a very personal concern. You call up all the images of the past and they are not comforting. I have had many people tell me that they are not apprehensive about being dead. They do worry about and fear "the dying." It is best to learn about the dying process when the information can be taken in without needing to apply it immediately. This gives you the opportunity to know the facts and form an attitude that will allow you to be well during the entire dying process.

This book is intended to uncover some of the mystery surrounding the dying process. It will correct the misconceptions you may have gotten from movies, television and books. This will lead all who approach this natural event to some degree of understanding. Armed with knowledge and with less fear you will be able to make reasonable and comforting decisions about where, how, and with whom death should occur. The people who continue to live must feel that the decisions that were made were the right ones for all concerned. This is absolutely essential for comfort and peace during the grieving process.

The Living End

We are wonderfully made. Our bodies are designed to stay in balance even though they are attacked by germs or injuries. Our bodies have built in armies to fight microbes and a repair system to heal damaged tissues caused by injury or just living. This battle to maintain our bodies in the best possible way continues as we enter the terminal phase of a disease. We need to know about the natural changes that do occur and then allow the body to do what it has been doing all our lives. Helping us be the best we can be. This will cause less discomfort and frustration, and it certainly is more economical. Nature has provided us with a wonderful system to ease us from a vital, active, well functioning body to the end of the life continuum.

As a nurse I have worked with dying people and their families in hospitals and in homes. I have seen suffering and fear eased when people learn about the natural progression of the human body during the dying process. Families, fortified with knowledge, have made decisions that benefited everyone. They have had the courage and confidence to confront the medical professional when that was necessary. They could demand that compassionate care, but not aggressive treatment, be given to the dying person.

Rita was such a person. She lived in New York City but returned to St. Louis because her mother, Virginia, was dying of cancer. Rita was a competent, self confident young woman, who had a successful career in New York. She was small and attractive and a "take control" kind of person. Faced with her mother's condition and her lack of knowledge all these attributes failed her. She chose to stay with her mother at the hospital so she was provided with a cot in Virginia's room.

I was called to do private duty for Rita's mother. Not because she needed extra care, but because Rita wanted the best possible care for her mother. I had taken care of Virginia's sister during her final days of life so I knew something about the family background and attitude. Since Rita spent her whole day with her mother, she and I had many conversations about her life with her mother and her life in New York. This allowed a rapport to develop between us so that she was able to trust my advice. I knew that she was committed to doing what was most humane for Virginia. When changes took place she asked about them, and I was able to step by step explain the functioning of the body at that point in the dying process. She believed me when I told her that certain things occur naturally during the dying process and that it is more comfortable for the person not to interfere. Supplied with information she was able to follow peacefully the changes in her mother. When Virginia's toes turned blue Rita understood that this was normal at this point and there was nothing to fear and no action was necessary. So she tranquilly watched and allowed herself to simply "be" with her mother during her final days. Rita was able to really share this dying process with Virginia.

Given the choice we would rather be eternally WELL. We don't have that choice. We do have the opportunity to learn to be well no matter where we are on the life-death continuum.

2. Spiritual Wellness

Elizabeth suffered a stroke. She was in her eighties and had lived an independent, active life before her stroke. There was residual paralysis after the stroke, so Elizabeth was no longer independent. She needed help bathing and dressing. After months of physical therapy, she was able to walk with a four pronged cane. She could also feed herself. However, her days of preparing meals for her husband were over. She could no longer do all the little household chores that she had taken pride and joy in doing for so many years. She was brave through all this and worked diligently with her physical therapist to regain as much use as possible from her useless left hand.

After almost nine months of struggle, Elizabeth suffered another stroke. It was obvious that she was very ill. As she lay in ICU she tried to fight her way back to living. Each day her family visited hoping that she could survive. The day came when her husband knew that she was tired of the fight and that she needed peace. With a great show of love, one evening before he left for the day, he said to her, "Sweetheart, I love you very much. I want you with me always, but if you need to go home to God I understand. I will miss you so much, but I will survive." After that he kissed her tenderly. Then with stooped shoulders, a slow gait, and a very sad face, he turned and walked out of the hospital. In the middle of the night he received the telephone call that informed him that his beloved wife had accepted his release. This was spiritual wellness. Elizabeth hung on to life for love of her husband and her husband was able to release her because of his great love.

Spiritual wellness deals with relationships. These relationships are with God, family, friends and yourself. When we talk about anger, conflict, self-esteem, intimacy, forgiveness, and love, we are talking about relationships. How we relate to ourselves and others affects our happiness and our peace of mind.

Spiritual wellness includes our relationship with a supreme being. It is important to be comfortable with this. You can not be really well until you develop this dimension. Spend some time each day sitting quietly just being with your creator.

We also need to be aware of our inner self. This is the part of us that is hidden deep within sometimes called the "real self." We want to discover who we are and what we want to accomplish.

To be really well we need to focus some times on our spiritual selves. In our society we concentrate on the material things in our lives-- things that we can see and hold and count. There is more to us than that, so much more. The dying person very often becomes consumed with thinking only of what is happening to the physical... to the body. There is so much to be gained by thinking about the spiritual realm and to develop this aspect to the fullest. Now is the time to hone relationships--to appreciate all those who have played a significant part in life. It can be a wonderful, joyful time.

In his book <u>Head First</u> Norman Cousins tells the story about a judge who was dying of cancer. The man had been known for his courage, determination and positive outlook. Now he had totally given up and was refusing to eat. His family could not understand his attitude and was devastated by his apathy. Norman Cousins visited the judge and explained to him what his lack of interest in life was doing to his family. He further told the judge that research showed that a negative attitude on the part of a patient could damage the health of the family. That day the judge changed. He resumed eating and taking an interest in life. Cousins goes on to say that the judge survived for several more weeks.

Once the judge understood that he was not the only one affected by his action, he was able to take an active part in living. He was also able to control the circumstances of his dying. Our goal in wellness is not to live forever, but to live fully. The clock and calendar are not the measure of our existance. The way we use our time, the meaning we invest in each minute, will be the final guage of how worthy and memorable a life is. Dying is not a tragedy. The tragedy is to die, never having discovered all of the possibilities and potentials in ou day to day living. Those who invest time and effort into positively affecting the lives of others will never really die because their influence has a ripple effect that goes on and on. How often do we quote our parents, grandparents and great grandparents in ordinary conversation? Relationships are powerful.

Many people never take time to think about who they are and why they are here. We are so busy with the "nuts and bolts" of living that we miss the subtle miracles that happen all around us. Watching a young child grow and develop is one small miracle after the other. When was the last time you watched the sunrise or the sunset? Have you ever marveled at how well your car works most of the time? Have you ever wondered about the fact that you think about things in concepts, but without conscious effort sentences come out of your mouth? There are so many wonderful, spiritual events happening around us that we so seldom appreciate. A person who is spiritually well and is dying can show those of us who are to "busy" to notice all the extraordinary, yet ordinary, things that we are missing.

The opportunity to share these things can only come when all members of the family can talk openly about dying. When the family is fearful about being open and honest, they miss many opportunities for closeness and sharing.

When Fred was in the hospital for the fourth time in one year, things were not going as well as the family had hoped. In the past Fred had responded well to chemotherapy, but this time he was very weak and the cancer was spreading. No one in the family had talked to him about their fears. It was a family that had a history of not discussing their emotions and feelings. Fred had been a widower for many years and had been independent and active. Now some decisions had to be made and his children did not know where to begin. No one knew for sure what Fred's physician had told him. To make matters worse the nursing staff didn't know how to handle the situation. Everyone knew that there was stress and tension, but they all backed away from trying to make a positive move. It was simply that no one knew what to do. At this point, I was made aware of the situation. One evening before Fred's daughter left after visiting, she and I entered his room. I explained to Fred that I wanted to talk with him. I then asked how he thought his treatment was going. He was very open with me about his condition. He informed me that he was aware that his condition was deteriorating and that death was approaching. We then discussed what he wanted his treatment to be in the future. He was able to let his daughter know that while he wanted to remain in his home as long as possible, he did not want to be an impossible burden to her or any other member of the family. Once there was open communication in this family they were able to live in peace with the knowledge that they could help Fred die according to his wishes.

To be spiritually well you want to be conscious of your purpose in life. Why are you here? What is your reason for being? You want to consider your relationship with God or higher power. All of us need time and space to worship our God. It is a need deep in the core of our being. In this materialistic world, we seldom take time to quietly sit and be with God. We can benefit from walking in the woods or anywhere in nature, just to get in touch with what is plain and simple and yet majestic and splendid.

In our relationships with others, few of us intentionally seek out and form meaningful friendships. We allow chance to place people in our path... people with whom to communicate. It is healthy to know your needs and seek those who can fill these needs. We also want those with whom we can share. Those special people tune into who we are and appreciate us. People travel all over the world searching for physical cures, but they don't make similar efforts to satisfy their need to love, share, play and be joyful.

In our society today, we are reluctant to make our needs known. It is so hard to ask for help. After Elizabeth's stroke, she was required to ask for many things that she handled for herself in the past. This was hard for her. It did allow her to grow. And it allowed those around her to show their love by helping.

It is not just meeting physical needs that is important. We each need someone to listen to us. To really hear not just the words, but to hear what we are saying with our hearts. We need someone to support us emotionally. To be ready to encourage us to get up when we fall. When our feelings are hurt, when we sense that others don't understand, we need someone to turn to who cares and has our best interest at heart. We need someone to challenge us emotionally. That special person who can tell us we do have what it takes to survive no matter what. That person who allows us to feel what we are feeling, but helps us get on with life. We also need someone with whom to play. Someone to make us laugh and see the humor in life. Someone who allows us to be carefree and joyful.

Forgiveness is an important part of spiritual wellness. As we live and relate to others we are sometimes hurt and suffer hurts from those we love. It is very often because of poor communications, but still the pain is there. It is essential that we forgive those who have hurt us. It is not always possible to contact each person personally. The person may have died, moved away, or we may not feel comfortable renewing a relationship with the offender. However, for our own peace of mind we must forgive. This can be a very healing event. When we carry around resentment, it is like a sore festering. The sore cannot heal until we forgive. Forgiveness does not mean that we accept the hurt and say that it was okay for the other person to hurt us. We don't have to approve of the offender's action. You simply visualize the person and tell him that you forgive him for the transgression. With that modest exercise the healing begins.

Barbara had been hurt by her husband's inattention for years. She was unhappy and was unable to find real contentment. She actually was punishing herself for her husband's actions, but she was not aware of this. When she was able to forgive her husband, the burden she had been carrying for years dropped from her and she was able to think of him without resentment. Forgiving is very healing.

The Living End

Those who are dying have a wonderful opportunity to think about the past. They can then make amends to those who will be left behind when death comes. This is a wonderful gift to give to those who will continue to live. When this forgiving is not done the survivors suffer unnecessary remorse and punishment.

Years after Rhonda's mother died she thought about what was left unsaid. She mourned the fact that she was not able to settle the differences between her mother and herself. She had cared for her mother during the final days of life, but they were not able to discuss the misunderstandings and forgive each other for these disagreements. With help from an understanding friend and after years of suffering, Rhonda was able to forgive her mother. She used imagery to picture her mother and ask forgiveness as well as giving forgiveness. It was a wonderful healing process for Rhonda, but it would have been so much better for both Rhonda and her mother if this could have taken place while the mother still lived.

3. Mental Wellness

Pattie was in her middle thirties and she was dying of cancer. Pattie had fought breast cancer for many years, but finally the disease had spread to other parts of her body. I took care of her in her home. She had had a chordotomy to relieve the constant pain of her disease. Chordotomy is a technique in which nerves are severed near the spinal cord to interrupt pain messages. The risk of the procedure is that it can cause paralysis below the point of severance. This happened to Pattie and therefore she was unable to move from her waist down. Despite her limitations this lady was spiritually and mentally well. There were many who cared for her that did not understand her. My supervisor thought that Pattie was in denial. I learned that it was not true. She was very aware of her condition and what the future held for her.

The Living End

Pattie was hard to get to know because she had experienced many skeptics. Many people who took care of her did not understand what she said. They assumed that they knew what she was trying to convey. As I became better acquainted with her, we talked about her condition and where she was headed. She told me that she had been rejected by a hospice program because she would not agree that she had less than six months to live. She felt that this was no way to "live." One day we were discussing her inability to walk. She told me that no one believed her, but she knew that she would walk again. Then she challenged me and asked if I believed her. I assured her that I did believe her. I shall never forget the look on her face or her response. She said: "I may never walk again in this life, but I will dance in Heaven." I knew then that she was fine. I could learn from her and I did.

To be mentally well implies more than the ability to think and act reasonably. It involves learning to adjust and adapt to the little aggravations and upsets that occur each day. We must be aware that along with the roses of life there are thorns. When these upsets come along a good question to ask is: "Will this matter a month from now, a week from now, or even tomorrow." Sometimes we waste energy on events that really don't matter. We want to cope with each problem as it arises and then let go of it.

This can be a reality even when the body is in less than perfect working condition. "Cope with problems as they arise." The problem with most of us is that we are burdened by "what ifs." We do not live in the moment, but spend our energy trying to solve problems that might happen. This is not reasonable and it is not even possible. You can't change a flat tire if it is not yet flat. You can change a not flat tire with the fear that it might go flat, but that is foolish. So is fretting about "what ifs." The mentally well person lives in the moment and savors what is here and now. This becomes very important to the dying person. The future is uncertain, so the ability to really "be" today takes on great significance. This is certainly possible when you concentrate on what is happening-- the sun that is shining, the good feeling that you are experiencing, the pleasant taste of the food that you can eat, the encouraging greetings from the people who love you. These are possible. These are present. These make ì you mentally well.

Many times when a person is ill they hand their body over to the physicians to treat as they see fit. Mentally well people take responsibility for themselves and make their own decisions. They learn what they can about the possible treatments and outcomes and then decide for themselves what route they chose to go. The problem with the phrase: "I trust my doctor to do what is best" is that you have given away responsibility for your own body. You are the only one who knows what is best for you and therefore you are the one who should be making the decisions. Ask questions. Read books. Visit the library. You can and should become an expert on the disease that is affecting you.

As you study you will find that the experience is exhilarating. It is always fun to learn. Your mind will be in control. You will open yourself to new and exciting experiences. The day when the doctor was the only one to know about disease and its treatment is over.

After a person is diagnosed with a disease, the tendency is to become that disease. You hear phrases like: "I am a heart patient," "I am a cancer victim," "I have AIDS." These people then become their disease. When they walk down the street they expect people to know that they are a heart disease or they are cancer. They wear this disease like a cloak, covering all that they really are. Their thought process revolves around them as disease. They may talk about "their disease" as they would talk about the prize that they won in a tournament. It becomes their trophy. They allow themselves to be swallowed by their diagnosis. This is not healthy. This is not being mentally well. In his workshops and books, Bernie Segal talks about people who survive because they do not become their disease. They tolerate what is happening to their bodies, but they continue to be who they are. Many times they spend more time appreciating being fully who they are. As a visiting nurse, I cared for just such a person.

Alma was in her seventies and she lived alone. When I read her medical history I was amazed that she could care for herself without daily help. She had heart disease so advanced that she was no longer a candidate for by-pass surgery, she suffered from diabetes that was difficult to control, and she was almost totally blind. As I prepared to visit her the first time, I expected to find a frail woman who had difficulty getting around and who would list her many ailments to me. When I stood on her doorstep and knocked on her door I was ireeted by a neat, clean lady with a happy smile on her face. I told her I was there to see Alma. To my great surprise she said she was Alma and then invited me in. Her house was immaculately clean and pleasantly though simply decorated. She chatted about the hot day and world events. When I asked how she was doing she said: "Oh! I can't complain." And all the time I cared for her she didn't. My next big surprise came when she told me that she wanted to learn how to test her own blood sugar. Despite the fact that she had limited vision, that little lady did learn how to do the procedure. She measured it accurately two times a day.

Alma did not wear her diagnosis as a cloak. She did not carry it around like a trophy. She put her disease on the shelf and only took it out to deal with when she needed. Her illnesses did not control her. She controlled them. She was very mentally well even though her body had problems.

In his book <u>Man's Search For Meaning</u>, Viktor Frankl tells about his work in a concentration camp during World War II. He was a psychiatrist in Germany before becoming a prisoner in the camp. He noticed that some robust, healthy looking people were not able to survive prison, but frail, fragile individuals managed to live through their ordeal. As ì a scientist he was intrigued. He learned that the difference was that: "--everything can be taken from a man but one thing: the last of the human freedoms-to choose one's attitude in any given set of circumstances, to choose one's own way." No matter what happens to you, it can destroy you or it can make you strong. The choice is yours.

Frankl said that we have choices to make every hour, every day even in a concentration camp, even as a dying person. You need to decide if you are going to submit to the powers that threaten to rob you of your self, your dignity, your inner freedom. You decide if you will "become the plaything of circumstances, renouncing freedom and dignity," or you choose to take control and make decisions for yourself.

Frankl discovered that when people found meaning in what they must endure they could persevere. He states that each situation is unique and therefore the meaning for each individual will need to be discovered by that person. He sums it up in this way:

When a man finds that it is his destiny to suffer, he will have to accept his suffering as his task - his single and unique task. He will have to acknowledge the fact that even in suffering he is unique and alone in the universe. No one can relieve him of his suffering or suffer his place. His unique opportunity lies in the way in which he bears his burden.

This is the challenge. The opportunity to be the best you can be with the reality presented to you. No other can do this for you. You have the chance to teach those you love how you need to be treated--what you want them to do for you, and how they can go on living when you are gone. Only you can do this for them. If you don't do it for them, it will not be done. You as a dying person cannot afford to be passive. There is too much work for you to do.

4. Emotional Wellness

We go through life busy with many things. We want to be happy. We want to be successful. What is success? What is happiness? Society measures success by your bank account, your house, the neighborhood you live in, and your automobile. And how do we measure happiness? Society dictates that if you are successful, you are happy. If that is true, many of us are in trouble. Fortunately, it is not true. Emotional wellness allows us to be successful and happy with very little material accumulation.

Each of us is different. We are needed in this world for a particular job. Something that we alone are able to accomplish. Many of us fail to discover our uniqueness and thus chase through life after someone else's mission. The secret is to find out who you are at the core of your being. To learn what unique things you have to offer to the world. When you discover this you will be able to do what will make you content and emotionally well.

The problem of having a blurred image of who we are begins when we are infants. We first think that everyone is an extension of ourselves. As we grow, we learn that we are all individuals, but we learn who we are from what others say to us, what others say about us, how they treat us, and the names they call us. We develop our self-image from those who are around us. When the majority of this input is positive we grow up with a good picture of who we are. When the feedback is mostly negative our self-image suffers. One way or another the day comes when, as adults, we must look at this self-image and decide for ourselves if the labels match who we really are now.

Richard Carson, in <u>Taming Your Gremlin</u>, describes an exercise that can help you identify any areas in your life that may be causing you confusion. He suggests that you draw the floor plan of the house that you lived in when you were between the ages of 3 and 7. Try to actually feel how you felt then and try to remember as many things as possible from each room. Take your time with this even spacing it over several days. After you finish with the floor plan try to answer the following: In this house what did you learn about the expression of love, hugging and kissing, causing people pain, who makes family decisions, how sadness and joy are expressed, trust and honesty, how men and women are, how smart, athletic, or creative you are, how lovable you are, and how likable you are.

After answering these questions, go back over your answers and notice if the things you learned at this young age are still driving your opinion about yourself. It could be that it is time for a change. Remember that your parents made choices about things for their life style and for their home. That was their right. It is also your right to make choices for yourself and for your home. It is not a matter of what is right or what is wrong. It is simply, but significantly, a matter of choice.

Truly emotionally well people have a capacity to feel deeply and to experience a wide variety of feelings. Feelings are not only the sensations you experience through the skin. Feelings are a state of mind, your connection with the world and other people, your interpretation of events around you. Most of us limit our awareness of our feelings. When I present workshops on wellness, I ask the participants to name some common feelings. Four out of five feelings named are negative feelings. They will identify anger, sadness, fear, loneliness, and being mad before they will remember happiness. Well people will recognize their positive feelings and appreciate them.

It is important to be aware of a wide variety of feelings. There are over 270 feelings that can be identified and yet most of us will label feelings only by the major categories such as anger. It is better to look deeper and recognize the real feelings of frustration, disappointment, or any other feelings. This will make a big difference in the way we react. If we think we are angry then we feel victimized, but if we feel frustrated then we can look for a positive act to alleviate the strain.

There are many ways to begin to recognize your real feelings. First make as long a list as you can of different feelings. Then several times a day stop and identify the feelings that you are experiencing at that moment. It may seem difficult at first, but with practice you will soon be an expert at accurately naming your feelings.

It is very important to appropriately identify feelings because that influences how we respond and thus it gives us more control over what we do. Really well people are willing to experience many different feelings. They express a wide range of appropriate feelings and this makes it comfortable for others to be with them. They are true to themselves and this gives them an aura of peace which is nice to be around.

Many people limit their feelings to a narrow range in order to protect themselves from bad feelings. Unfortunately, this also prevents them from benefiting from good feelings. The big problem is that people confuse experiencing emotions with expressing them. You may be mad at someone because they insulted you. You can recognize this feeling without needing to punch them in the nose. You can notice your feeling and decide that the speaker is not worthy of your attention. This would be the well way to handle the situation. You do not have to deny that you are mad in order to avoid the punch. Denying how you feel is not necessary; in fact, it is not recommended. Learn to be very aware of your feelings. Develop a vocabulary that includes all the subtle shades of your emotional experience. Take control of how you respond. You can do this, it just takes practice.

Since anger is such an important emotion we should spend some time on it. Anger is not a reflex. We do not automatically become angry the same way we jerk a hand away from a hot surface. It is an unpleasant emotion that we choose as a response to an event. No one can be made angry against their will. You may not always be consciously aware that you are choosing anger. You may feel uncomfortable and act to relieve this discomfort by shouting at your neighbor or storming out of a room and slamming the door.

Anger is a feeling; it is not an action. It is not wrong or incorrect to feel angry. How you choose to act in response to the angry feeling can be good or bad. When your boss unjustly criticizes you, you can use your anger in very constructive ways like working more diligently. You may react negatively by making unpleasant jokes about that boss. The positive reaction will make you feel better and vindicated, but the negative reaction will leave you feeling worse.

The problem with nurturing anger is that it grows and grows so that you become angry about everything. You think that everyone is against you, you become irritable and aggressive, you try to blame others for everything that happens even when no one is to blame, because sometimes things just happen. Angry people spend their energy in trying to defeat those that they see as their enemies. It can be very destructive.

Anger can be difficult to overcome. The angry people begin to enjoy exploding in a rage. They perceive that they are justified in holding grudges. The pleasant discharge of anger reinforces this negative response to anger. You can learn to control your habit by first

The Living End

becoming aware of it and then deciding that you want to change. After that you choose positive actions when you feel anger. It will take time, but it will be worth the effort.

Kubler-Ross identifies anger as one of the stages after a terminal diagnosis. Some people channel this anger in positive ways. They channel the energy towards being as well as they can be for as long as they can and learn all they can about their disease and what will happen. Other people choose to become withdrawn and vent negative actions against those who have not received such a diagnosis. This is a good example of choosing to use a feeling to make you better or to make you worse.

The dying person can refine their emotional wellness. They have the opportunity to help their care-takers to tune into their own wellness. There are, however, several emotional situations that are distinctive to the dying process. One that is often difficult to deal with is that of detachment. This is a letting go of those things that were of interest to the person in the past. This is often seen in the elderly and those who are chronically ill for a long time before death. It can begin to occur as long as a year before death occurs. In the young or those acutely ill, the manifestation of detachment will be shorter - sometimes weeks, sometimes days, and sometime only hours.

The dying person gradually loses concern for the ordinary things of life along with their special interests. You will notice that they ask to watch television less. They may cease reading the newspaper or other material. You will find them sitting or lying and simply staring off into space. The detachment of a dying person is similar to a person getting ready to go on vacation. Your attention is focused on packing and planning your trip. You have diminished concern for the events around you. It is also very similar to when you resign or retire from a job. Suddenly the people around you talk about what will happen with the business and their future, but you know you are not a part of this so you just tune them out and think your own thoughts.

This detachment is very hard for the family to understand and accept. They keep trying to drag the dying person back to their world. They want them to show the same interest in things that they have exhibited in the past. The family unconsciously believes that if they are involved in family matters they will not be very sick, that they will not die. It is a form of denial or a way of coping by the family.

Mona had a stroke and was not expected to live. She was alert, but unable to speak well. Her family gathered around her bedside and with excited, rapid speech told her about the grandchildren and the events in the family. Mona lay there. Her face was a mask. You could feel the sentences hanging in the air. You could sense the desperation of her children as Mona failed to respond with the same intense interest that she has always displayed. They didn't know. They didn't want to know that she was "packing her bags" for her trip into death.

Mona's family didn't appreciate it at the time, but she was helping them to prepare for their lives without her. Her body was still with them, but her spirit was letting go and giving those she loved a chance to slowly let go of her. It is so much more peaceful when family members can accept the period of detachment and enjoy those times when the dying person can be fully engaged with familiar events. As they acknowledge what is happening, the family can then share with the dying person how they perceive things. This way each can learn from the other.

People face the reality of their own death in different ways. It may appear to others that the dying person is denying his prognosis. You should ask the person about his views on their prognosis. They may be processing the situation in their heads and they don't have a need or they don't want to share this process with anyone.

When I cared for Sara in her home, her physician said that she had less than two weeks to live. Her family had not discussed this with her. They thought that she was not aware of her prognosis, so they asked me to talk with her.

Sara had worked as a volunteer in one of the large hospitals. She was familiar with illness and dying. She knew about the hospice programs in the area, but she chose to live her last days at home with as little change in the family routine as possible. When I asked her about her perception of what was happening to her, she said in a strong, confident voice, "I think you can talk too much about this. I know I am dying and there is nothing to be said about it." She was not denying her condition, she was accepting the best way she could. A few days later as she struggled with walking from her bed to the bathroom, she looked at me with sorrow written across her face and said: "This is not quality life." This brave lady embraced death with eagerness and tranquillity a few days later.

There is a cycle of fear and peace that dying people experience as they work out their adjustment to their new status. It is interesting that these dual feelings of peace and fear are also observed in the animal kingdom. At first the periods in the cycle are dramatic and long, lasting for days or weeks. The period of fear will be intense with illogical thoughts and anxiety. The person may become restless and engage in constant motion. They will frantically investigate their condition, hoping to find a new answer. It is both reasonable and recommended to get a second option, but to travel all over the world seeking a better diagnosis may not be in the best interest of anyone. Some people will spend hours in the library reading every book they can find on the subject and listen to every person who will talk to them. They research the topic as though it had nothing to do with them, however they almost insist that there is a complete recovery in the future for them.

Then there will be a period of peace and calm. There will be intense quiet and tranquillity lasting the same length of time as the fear. During this time the storm has abated and it seems that the dying person has forgotten their disease. Once again they will enjoy life, proceeding with the normal daily routine as though nothing had happened. This is a wonderful time for the family, because relationship problems can be resolved.

Gradually the peaks and valleys of peace and fear will become less intense and the period of fear will be shorter, until there is final peace and adjustment. This cycle of peace and fear is present even in the acutely ill or victims of accidents. It is harder to observe because there is so much activity around the person that often no one notices the emotional status of the dying person.

With knowledge about the dying process the transition to peace and adjustment can be attained with minimum pain from the fear period. Part of the fuel that fires the passion of the fear period is the lack of knowledge about what will happen to the body, how the person will feel about this, and how the family will react. Certainly no one of us knows for sure how we will react to any event in the future, but with an understanding of what is likely to happen we can be prepared.

5. Physical Wellness

Physical wellness is characterized by the ability to do what you want to do, when you want to do it. You have the energy to act throughout the day without extreme fatigue. You have the strength and endurance to meet the challenges that you encounter. Each person has their own definition for what is physical wellness. Some of this has to do with age. My 95 year old father believes he is physically well when he is able to go though a day without unusual pain and when he is able to move about his house without falling. A 25 year old person would consider this level of activity very limiting. So each of us has our own expectation for what physical wellness is to us.

We all agree that physical wellness involves the four elements of nutrition, exercise, relaxation, and play. You want to plan your day so that you have the opportunity to fill your need for each of these elements. This is what health care is. The Tubesings say: "Health care is something you do every day. It's not something to be delivered... it's to be acted out." How you treat your body will determine how your body will treat you. When you allow yourself an adequate balance of the four elements of physical wellness, you experience that healthy glow that all of us appreciate.

For the dying person, physical wellness is not a possibility. They can enjoy some of the benefits of physical wellness, but they have limits. It is important to have a good working knowledge of what will happen physically to the dying person, because knowing the possibilities will help them prepare for what is expected.

The next five chapters will deal with each body system separately. Keep in mind that the body does work as a unit so one system can affect the others. We are all built the same, but we are all different. That is why some of us are allergic to certain products, while others can enjoy them without problems. Because we are different, there will be individual differences in the way our bodies react to the dying process. Expect similarities, but allow for differences as you proceed through the systems of the human body.

The Circulatory System

The heart has so much emotion attached to it that it is difficult to appreciate its clinical significance. There are songs written about the affairs of the heart. There are expressions like: "Have a heart," " he is heartless," and "think with your heart not your head." And we have cupid with the arrow through a heart and all the Valentine's day sentiment. It is no wonder then when we try to discuss the human heart as a pump, it becomes challenging to disassociate the metaphor from reality. We have this underlying belief that when something goes wrong with the heart you are doomed. We think we are more seriously ill than with a disease of any other part of the body. Maybe this is why there is so much research concerning heart disease and why there are numerous treatment modalities for the many identified heart diseases. Anyone who has ever had chest pain has experienced how quickly you are whisked into intensive care and put through hordes of tests. It is because of the "if we can name it we can treat it" mentality that exists with heart disease. During this ordeal the person is left with little information, but with the feeling that he must be in very bad condition. More reason and less panic in called for here. Remember, the heart is a pump.

Overview of the Anatomy and Physiology of the Heart and Blood Vessels

The heart is a pump with four chambers. It could be considered as two pumps joined together. The heart is located in the middle of the chest between the breast bone and the spinal structure. It is because of this location between two bony structures that cardiac massage is possible. It is interesting to note that all major organ are protected by bony structures. The right border of the heart lies along the right border of the breast bone. The left border of the heart stick out past the left border of the breast bone. The heart is tilted so that the left side rides higher in the chest than the right side. The heart weighs less than a pound and is the size of a person's fist. A baby's fist is small and their heart is small. As we grow our fists get bigger and so do our hearts. The heart begins beating long before birth, sometime around the fourth week after fertilization, and continues until death. It is a paradox that it works all the time and yet rests after each beat. The purpose of this pump is to move blood through a closed system of vessels.

The heart wall is made of three layers. The outer layer or sac is the pericardium. The middle layer, called the myocardium, is a special type of muscle different from all other muscles in the body. This special muscle allows each chamber to contract as a unit so that blood is forced out of the chamber all at once. The inner layer is a delicate lining known as the endocardium.

The inside of the heart consists of four chambers. There are two on the top called atria and two on the bottom known as ventricles. The muscle walls of the ventricles are much thicker than the atria because there has to be enough force to push the blood through the lungs and throughout the body. The ventricle wall on the left is thicker than the ventricle wall on the right side. Since the right side simply pumps blood through the lungs it requires less muscle power than pumping blood all the way down to the toes as the left side of the heart has to do.

The heart is divided by a thick wall into right and left sides. This thick muscle wall contains the electrical conduction system for the heart. The impulses that cause the heart to contract are in this structure. The heart is unique in that its rate is controlled from within the heart itself. There is the "pacemaker" in the right atrium called the sinoatrial (SA) node which sends out impulses that causes the heart muscle to contract. The heart can actually be taken out of the body and it will continue to beat. Messages from outside the heart can stimulate it to beat faster or slower, but these messages must go through the SA node.

Valves separate the atria and ventricles. Valves also separate the ventricles from the vessels leading away from the heart. The function of the valves is to allow blood to flow in one direction only. The valves in the atria open to allow the blood to be pumped into the ventricles. Then these valves snap shut and the valves leading into the vessels open to permit the blood to be ejected from the ventricles. After the ventricles contract forcing all of the blood out of them, the valves snap shut. It is this snapping action of the valves that is heard with the stethoscope. Since two valves work at the same time it takes strategy to hear just one snap shut. This is why a listener will place the stethoscope over different places on the chest. It takes an experienced ear to be able to separate the sounds and determine if a valve is sealing properly.

The blood, from the body, enters the right atrium. It is then pumped into the right ventricle; from there it is pumped into the lungs where it picks up oxygen and gives up carbon dioxide. The oxygenated blood is returned to the heart and dumped into the left atrium, which pumps it into the left ventricle. The blood is then pumped throughout the body to bring oxygen and nutrients to the cells and to collect the waste products of cell activity.

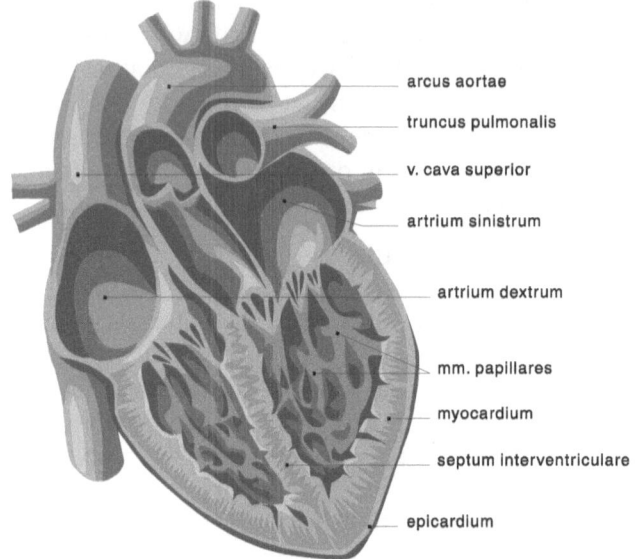

Figure 1: The Human Heart

When the blood leaves the heart to supply the body, some of this blood ì goes to the heart muscle itself. The vessels, that supply the heart muscle with blood, are known as coronary vessels. They are called this because the vessels form sort of a crown around the outside of the heart. If one of these vessels becomes blocked, the person experiences a heart attack. More about that later.

The two atria contract at the same time and then the two ventricles contract at the same time. There is a very short pause after the ventricles contract, before the atria contraction begins again. It is the contraction of the left ventricle that is felt as a pause and which is measured when taking a blood pressure. The blood vessels are a closed circuit. The vessels that lead away from the heart are called arteries and they have a pause. The vessels that lead back to the heart are recognized as veins; they sometimes have valves. The arteries and veins are joined by a network of capillaries.

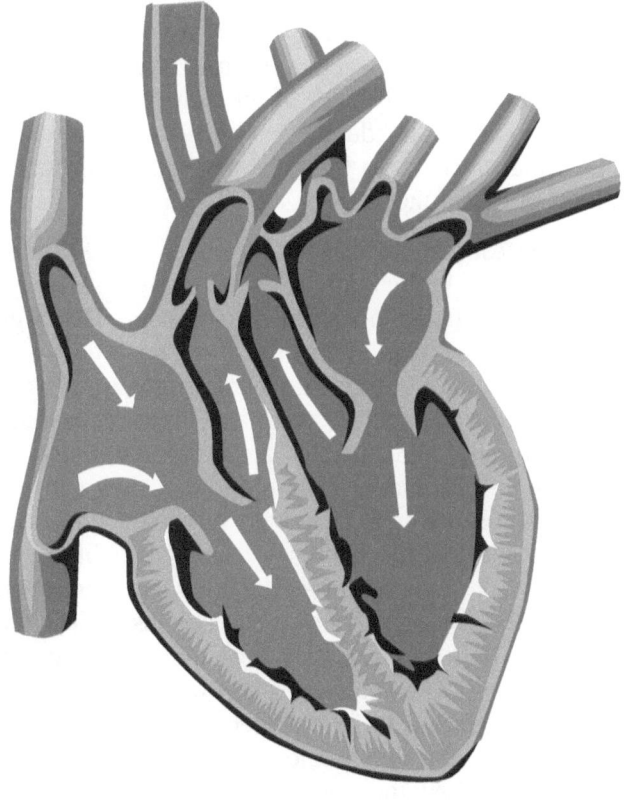

CARDIAC CYCLE
Figure 2: Cardiac Cycle

The vessels are made alike with three layers or coats. The outer layer is fibrous and allows the vessels to remain open instead of collapsing with each pause, however, the veins have fewer fibers to allow them to collapse when cut. The middle coat is made of smooth muscle which permits the contraction and dilation of the vessels during normal functioning of the heart and vessels. The inner coat is a lining layer; in undamaged vessels it is smooth. The capillaries are made of only the lining layer; the walls are only one cell thick. Although they are only 1/25 of an inch in diameter, it is the capillaries that do the real work of supplying oxygen and nutrients to the cells and gathering waste products of cells function.

It has been estimated that there are over 62,000 miles of blood vessels in the body. The layout of the arteries, veins, and capillaries looks like a road map. The large artery leaving the heart, called the aorta, soon begins to branch into smaller arteries sending vessels in all directions, like the four or five lane highway leading out of a big city. The arteries get smaller and smaller until they are capillaries. The blood that they carry is bright red because it is rich with oxygen. From the capillaries the vessels become veins. The blood in them is dark red because the oxygen has been removed. The vessels that you can see just below the skin appear dark because they are veins with oxygen depleted blood. The veins get larger and larger, just as roads leading into a large city get bigger and bigger. The large vein that dumps blood into the right side of the heart is called the vena cava. A layout of the arteries and the veins show that the major vessels run pretty much side by side. It makes them look even more like the roads going into and out of the big cities.

The average heart rate of a healthy adult is 72 beats per minute. At rest, the heart pumps one gallon of blood per minute. However it can increase its output to five and one half gallons per minute during maximum activity. The brain always receives one and one third pints per minute regardless of physical activity.

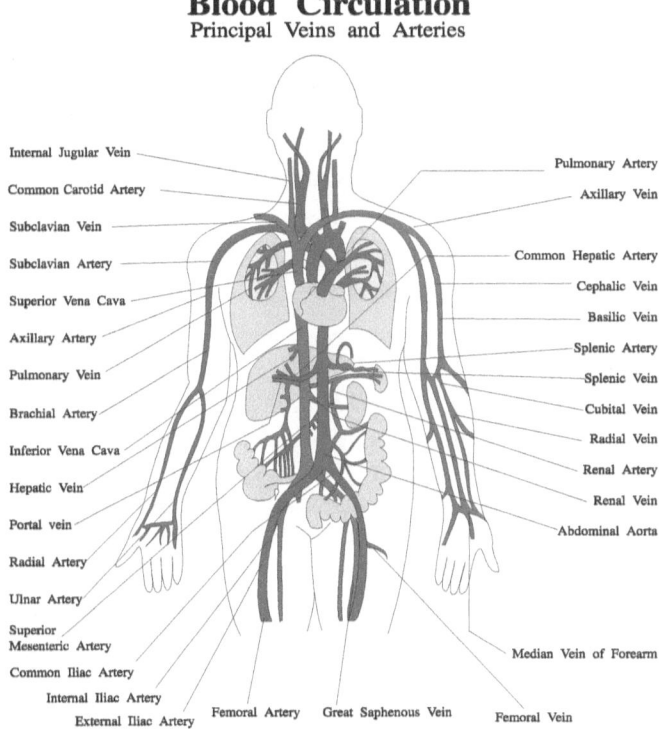

Figure 3: Circulatory System

The rate of the heart is regulated by the pacemaker inside the heart. This pacemaker receives impulses from the sympathetic and parasympathetic nerves systems which can affect the rate of the heart beat. This allows the heart to respond to the increased demand for blood during vigorous physical activity or emotional stress such as fright, sudden noises or nightmares.

The blood pressure is a measure of the most and least pressure exerted in the arteries. In an adult it is normally 120/80mmHg. It is important because if the pressure in the arteries remains high over many years there is damage to the smooth lining of the arteries. Blood pressure responds rapidly to external and internal influences such as fear, stress, and kidney malfunction. High blood pressure is known as the silent killer because there are no symptoms to indicate to a person that their blood pressure is elevated. It is only when the pressure is very high that some people will suffer from a headache.

When all is functioning normally, the heart pumps away keeping all our cells in a healthy environment. We never have to think about our next heart beat. We don't have to worry about our blood pressure or our heart rate. It is automatic. It is efficient. It is continuous. It only asks that we treat it right with good nutrition, good exercise, good sleep, relaxation, meditation and caring for and sharing with others. That isn't much to ask for what we get in return.

How the Dying Process Affects the System

The heart slows its activity during the dying process. It no longer pumps as forcefully. As a result of this, fluids begin to build up in the tissues. This swelling, or edema as it is known, is first seen in what is called the dependent parts, such as the feet, ankles, or back. Later there may be edema of the legs, hands, and arms.

At this point the circulation is also impaired. With less force of the heart beat, the blood flow to the extremities decreases. This results in a mottling of these extremities. This is a variable bluish discoloration of the skin. The toes are usually the first to become discolored, but sometimes there may be mottling of the finger tips as well. This mottling will slowly move up the extremities. As this occurs, the first discolored parts will become distinctly blue or even black. Along with the discoloration, the extremities become cold to the touch. At the time of death, the feet and lower legs may be totally blue or black and feel quite cold when touched. Even though these parts feel cold to you, the person does not sense coldness because the ability to feel hot and cold has been diminished. It is not necessary, in fact, it is not advisable to add external warmth as a comfort measure for the person.

Another manifestation of the less forceful pumping of the heart is congestion or fluid build up in the lungs. It is referred to as "the death rattle." It is sometimes feared that the person has developed pneumonia, as the fluid builds up in the lungs. More than likely it is congestion that results from greatly decreased circulation. Fluid usually collects in the lungs during the last two or three days, except in those persons whose primary condition is attributed to lung disease. Then the congestion will occur much earlier. The physiology of this is the same as the fluid build-up in the dependent parts, but there is also a slowing of circulation in the lungs themselves. This adds to the accumulation of fluids.

As the heart and circulation of blood in the dying person are slowing down the fluid build-up will be greater if the person is receiving intravenous fluids. This artificial fluid intake will cause an increased congestion of the lungs and collection of fluid in the abdomen. This causes great discomfort to the person.

Virginia had an abdomen that was quite enlarged with fluids. She was restless with discomfort. She was receiving intravenous fluids. Because she was in the dying process she was not able to handle these artificial fluids so they accumulated in her abdomen. One day the fluids began to infiltrate into the tissue around the vein where the needle, for the intravenous fluids, was inserted. This happens often during the dying process for two reasons. The body has difficulty handling the added fluids and the vessels begin to collapse. It was decided not to try to restart the intravenous fluids for Virginia. As a result of not having added fluids, the swelling in her abdomen decreased and she rested much more quietly.

Later Virginia's physician wanted to initiate clysis. This is a method of giving fluids just below the skin. Rita, in a gallant manner, demanded that no artificial fluids be given to her mother. She had to argue with the physician and even threaten to fire him if he insisted on giving fluids. This was not fair to her. It increased her anguish, but in the end she was able to spare her mother the unpleasant pain of fluids that her body could not manage.

You can request that artificial fluids be discontinued. This will free the person from intravenous tubing and needles, which are constraining. It will also eliminate the need for the painful procedure of restarting the intravenous fluids, which will become more frequent as the blood flow slows and the vessels tend to collapse. Giving intravenous fluids to the dying person causes more stress to everyone. Since it is not of benefit to the person, but merely adds to discomfort, it should not be done.

Many times the family has to take the initiative and ask that only true comfort measures be used. It is sad to relieve the person of the intravenous needle only after death has been pronounced.

Clara knew that she was dying. She had fought emphysema for many years. Now not only her lungs, but her heart was affected and she was tired of the fight. She told her family that she did not want any more treatments. Her family honored this request. She had no intravenous fluids. She did receive some medication to help her breathing and she was given oxygen. The family gathered at her bedside. It was a close family that had enjoyed many happy times together. They sat and chatted with each other. Sometimes Clara joined in, but most of the time she lay in her bed listening with a very contented smile on her face. Her eyes glowed when she talked about going home to Heaven. There was little struggle and little stress as Clara spent her final hours in peace with her family.

The heart rate is not an indicator of the dying process. In some people the rate and strength of the pulse will decrease gradually. In others there will be a cessation of breathing and then a slowing of the heart beat over a period of a minute or so. A person whose cause of death is due to heart disease may have an increasingly erratic heart beat until the heart stops completely. This erratic heart rate can last several days. There are medications that can be given to smooth out this irregular rhythm, but since it is causing no harm there is no need for this.

The blood pressure drops as the dying process progresses. Sometimes the drop is dramatic. Often it will go down slightly, then return to normal only to drop again. There are medications to stabilize this. They are useful in people who are experiencing shock or other treatable conditions, but as a normal event in the dying process, such changes should be allowed to happen naturally. Ultimately the drop in blood pressure will be low enough to effect the function of the kidneys. This will be discussed in the next chapter.

Some Primary Diseases of the Heart and Blood Vessels

There are numerous identified diseases of the heart. Many of them can be successfully treated for many years. The fact is that sooner or later we all die and if we have been treated for a certain disease for many years then that disease will probably contribute to death.

The Living End

A heart attack, or myocardial infraction, is one of the leading causes of death in the United States. This happens when one of the coronary arteries becomes blocked. When such a vessel is obstructed, there is no longer ì blood flow to that part of the heart muscle. This not only causes severe pain, it results in the area of the heart to die. If a very large area is damaged it will significantly interfere with adequate contraction of that part of the heart. The outcome of this is decreased blood flow from that part of the heart. If the right lower chamber is involved the flow to the lungs will decrease. Since that chamber is not emptying properly it will cause blood to back up into the right upper chamber and ultimately into the tissue of the body. If the blockage is on the left ventricle it will cause blood to back up in the lungs leading to congestion. Fluid will then leak into the lung space interfering with proper gas exchange. These conditions are termed congestive heart failure. When it is mild it can be effectively treated, but the time arrives when the heart tires of the struggle to maintain normal functioning. It is then time to let go.

The biggest problem initially with heart attack is the irregular heart beat that results from the sudden stop of blood flow to the heart muscle. The ventricles' rhythm can become so impaired that the heart just quivers rather than contracting normally. This is known as ventricular fibrillation. It is treatable, but while it continues, no blood will be leaving the heart. Therefore there is no circulation anywhere including the heart muscle. If nothing is done to correct this it will result in what is called ventricular standstill, which means all heart activity stops. A person can tolerate this for only about four minutes before irreparable damage is done to the body.

After several heart attacks there will be so much damage to the heart that it can no longer sufficiently pump blood to the lungs and body. This produces cardiac shock or pump failure. The death rate from this is very high (80%).

The valves in the heart may become diseased and no longer close properly. This may occur after a serious infection such as rheumatic fever or endocarditis. The damage to the valves will impair proper function. Any of the valves can be involved. There could be scarring on the valve causing it to be stiff and therefore unable to open normally, thus impeding blood flow. The diseased valves may fail to close tightly causing blood to flow back into the chamber it has just left. All of these conditions prevent normal blood flow and thus normal oxygenation of the tissues. When the damage is slight the person may need to decrease usual activity, but they can continue to live relatively unencumbered with restrictions. If the valve damage is great normal activity will be impossible. Then the damaged valves will need to be replaced or activity extremely limited.

Cardiomyopathy is a disease of the heart muscle. This is a disease that is not well known. Because it mimics other heart diseases, the diagnosis is usually made by the process of elimination. The person with this disease will experience congestive heart failure and uncontrollable irregular heart rates. The disease is classified as primary and secondary. The cause of primary cardiomyopathy is not known and the prognosis is poor. Secondary cardiomyopathy is caused by such things as infection, neurologic or neuromuscular diseases, exposure to chemicals, radiation or drugs, and nutritional disorders. This is the disease that can ultimately kill drug addicts and anorexics. This disease manifests itself in several forms. The left ventricle dilates, the wall between the ventricles enlarges and bulges into the right ventricle, the wall between the ventricles enlarges and narrows the opening out of the left ventricles into the aorta. These can all be treated, but the person will lead a restricted lifestyle at best. The possibility of sudden death is a reality with which these people must learn to live.

In the movie Beaches, Heather develops Cardiomyopathy. She is young and enjoying a career as an attorney when the disease strikes. The movie shows how difficult it is to try to live with the threat of death in your prime. She states that she is not ready to face death and she struggles with her anger. The viewer can certainly appreciate her dilemma. When the diagnosis of cardiomyopathy is made then the situation is not a movie. It is real.

Atherosclerosis is most often the consequence of high blood pressure over a long period of time. There does not seem to be one single cause of high blood pressure; known in medical circles as hypertension. There is some wear and tear on the vessels in certain areas because of the turbulent flow of blood around corners and at forks in the vessels as they branch. But normally the blood flows through the vessels without damaging the lining of the vessels. If the blood strikes the wall with greater than normal force in the area where a vessel takes a sharp turn or branches, damage to the wall of that vessel can result. Once there is a rough place on the lining wall it is a target for platelets to gather. These platelets stick to the injured area and invite other platelets and cholesterol to adhere to the spot. This continues to narrow the opening causing a decrease in blood flow to the area beyond the formation. Ultimately several things could happen. The vessel will become completely blocked off, a traveling piece of material in the blood, like a small clot, will become wedged in the narrowed vessel, or a piece of the material will break off and travel to some other area and then become lodged in a vessel. In all these situations blood flow is stopped to a part of the body. It will cause pain. If it is a large vessel that is affected in a vital organ system, like the brain, the heart, the kidneys, or the lungs, it could cause sudden death.

The vessel wall could become very thin. This is often caused by hypertension also, but sometimes a person is born with a thin spot on a vessel wall. After a time, which is not definite, the vessel wall will bulge out forming an aneurysm. This is like a balloon filled with blood. They can form slowly over many years or they can materialize suddenly. The danger with this is that at some time it will rupture causing a life-threatening hemorrhage. Many times the presence of these aneurysms are not known until after rupture.

It has been well documented that lifestyle can be a big factor in causing hypertension and heart disease. There is no longer any question that smoking, chronic stress, diets high in saturated fats and limited physical exercise contribute to diseases of the heart and blood vessels. In his book <u>Reversing Heart Disease</u>, Dean

Ornish presents research showing that not only does a wellness lifestyle decrease your risks of these diseases, it can also reverse damage that has begun.

The Kidneys

Sam had been battling cancer for many months. His family was told that he was going to die soon. He was at home and although he had some pain and discomfort, he was able to move about with help. The day came when getting out of bed was too much of a burden for him. His wife noticed that his urine output was slowly becoming less. She also observed that it was a darker color with an offensive odor. As the time passed, Sam began to ask questions that didn't make sense. He talked to people that weren't present. Sometimes he talked to his dad who had been dead for several years. Then the periods of sleep began to increase. He was now resting so quietly his wifely would creep into the room to convince herself that he was still breathing. In just less than two days he peacefully slipped into death. No struggle. No moaning. No pain.

Overview of Anatomy and Physiology

Although the kidneys are small, they have a vital function. They remove waste products, toxins, and water from the body. They also maintain a normal concentration of sodium, potassium and chlorides. These are all very important activities. If the kidneys fail to maintain this proper balance and the condition is not remedied, the person will die.

The Living End

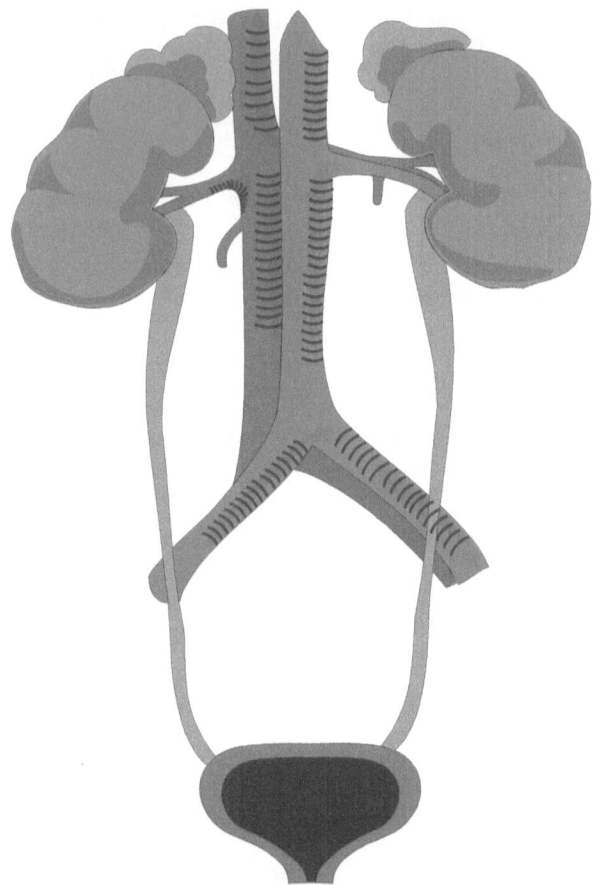

Figure 4: The Kidneys

The kidneys are four and one half inches long, two and one half inches wide, and one and one half inches thick. They are shaped like lima beans and are located in the back just above the waist, on either side of the spine. Although we have two kidneys, a person can survive normally with only one regularly functioning kidney.

The kidneys are made up of microscopic tubes called tubules which fold back and forth much like the coils in a car radiator. Thousands of feet of these tubules are packed into the small area of the kidneys. The blood vessels enter the kidney and pass by these tubules at the rate of 50 gallons per day. That means that two and a fourth pints of blood are pumped through the kidneys each minute. As the blood rushes through the kidneys, water and solid material called solutes contained in the blood are filtered out of the vessels into the tubules. This is accomplished because there is a difference in

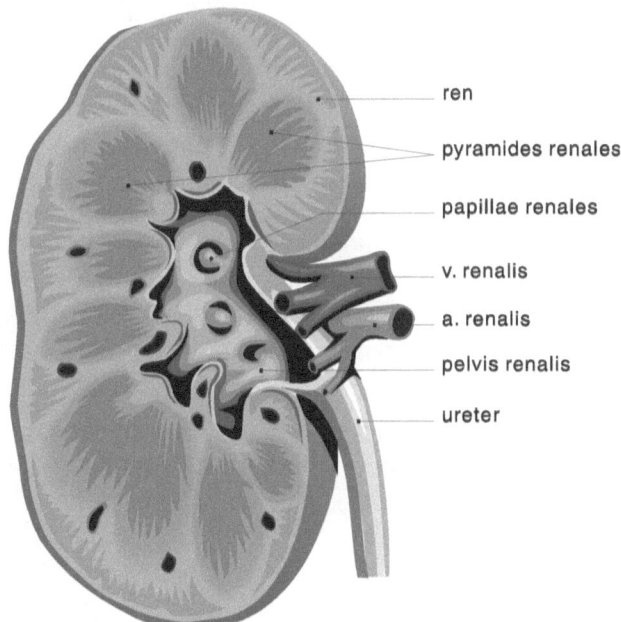

Figure 5: The Kidney Interior

pressure between the vessel and the tubule which is porous. As the material in the tubule moves along, the solutes that the body needs, such as sodium and potassium as well as some of the water, are returned to the blood. This allows the body to maintain its delicate body chemistry. The blood then flows out of the kidneys and continues its journey around the body to once again collect waste and toxin to return to the kidney. In the meantime, the kidney now has the ingredients to form urine. This urine will flow into the ureters on its way out of the body. The kidneys only produce two to three pints of urine each day, but these tiny filtering tubules in the kidneys are busy night and day deciding what solid materials to return to the body and how much fluid is needed to maintain a healthy fluid balance.

The other parts of the urinary system are the two ureters, which are small tubes about ten inches long that join the kidneys to the bladder. The bladder is a collapsible bag that holds urine. It is simply a reservoir. The urethra is a small tube whose function it is to transport urine outside the body from the bladder. In the male, it also transports reproductive fluid from the body.

Each of these structures can be affected by diseases. During the dying process the kidneys begin to slow down their function just as other organ systems do.

The Living End

How the Dying Process Effects this System

Blood pressure is a very important factor in the functioning of the kidneys. If the blood pressure drops because of disease or trauma outside the kidney, it will reduce the effectiveness of the filtering in the tubules. But if there is disease in the kidney causing a reduction in proper filtering, the blood pressure can either increase or decrease depending on the disease process. When the blood pressure drops very low, there is no longer enough force to move the waste, toxins, and water into the tubes. This allows the blood to return to the body without the waste and toxins being removed. It can also allow too much circulating fluid, causing an increased load on the heart, or allow fluid to filter out into the tissue of dependent parts such as the back, legs, arms or buttocks. This causes the whole body to function below normal thus making the person less alert and/or restless. Since all the blood moves through the kidneys many times an hour, it does not take long for the ill effects of poorly functioning kidneys to become noticeable.

The signs of poorly functioning kidneys are a decrease in the amount of urine that is expelled. The urine that is made will be concentrated giving it a very dark color and an unpleasant odor. The person will become less alert and confused. Ultimately, coma will result. In the dying process, this is seen about twenty-four to forty-eight hours before death. It may be longer than this if the kidneys are the primary source of disease.

At the time that the kidney function shows signs of decreasing, the medical professional may try to force the kidney into increased activity. They ì attempt this by rapidly giving intravenous fluid reasoning that if more fluid is flowing through the kidneys they will function more ì adequately. So by increasing the fluid in the blood there will be ì an increase of fluid flowing through the kidneys. This procedure is very uncomfortable for the patient and will not help in the final analysis because the failure of the kidney is simply a symptom of the dying process... not something that can be helped by increased fluid volume.

The natural way can be the most merciful way. As the patient becomes ì less alert they tend to rest more peacefully. It seems to be nature's way of easing a person into death without stress and struggle. I have seen quite peaceful deaths when the normal dying process is allowed to proceed through it's natural course.

Charles was diagnosed with cancer of the kidney. Although he accepted ì treatment with chemotherapy, he made the decision to make a living ì will. He instructed his wife, his physician, his lawyer, and his minister that he did not want his dying prolonged. His Living Will was very specific that he wanted relief from pain, but no other treatment ì including intravenous therapy.

Charles had nursing care in the home around the clock. When I first took care of him he was able to move about some. I remember taking him for a visit to his physician my first week of work. Even then his appetite was poor and I was instructed to encourage him, but not to force him to eat. After about ten days he was completely bed fast and consuming less than a baby.

The home atmosphere was wonderful. Charles' bed was in the area of the house just off the kitchen. This area had probably been the dining space, but now it was where Charles spent his time. I remember the family continuing with their normal activity around him and including him in the conversation. Even after he slipped into unconsciousness he was included.

One Sunday, Charles' parents were visiting for the afternoon. His dad stepped over to the bed, put his hand on Charles' shoulder and said to him: "Son, I love you so much. I am going to miss you, but I know you need to go." Two days later Charles died. He died peacefully as he had requested.

Some Primary Disease of the Kidneys

There are several diseases that can ultimately cause death even with medical treatment. This is not necessarily a failure it is just the way things are. No one is to blame.

There can be cancer of the kidney or the bladder. There are treatments for these, but the cancer may not be diagnosed in the early stages, it may be a rapid growing cancer, or it may have started in some other area and moved into the kidney or bladder.

There can be a chronic infection of any of the structures in the urinary system that can cause damage to the normal tissue. The normal tissue then no longer functions adequately so normal removal of waste, toxins and water is decreased. As the normal tissue is replaced by damaged tissue the whole system is compromised. Chronic infection can also cause scar tissue to form thus making the inside diameter of the tubes smaller and stiffer. This will slow down the flow of urine and other fluids.

The vessels inside the kidney may become stiff and hard. This is often caused by prolonged high blood pressure, smoking or other unhealthy lifestyle activities. When the vessels are hard and stiff they can no longer filter the blood sufficiently.

Any of these conditions can continue long enough to be the primary cause of death. Sometimes transplant or dialysis is prescribed, but these are not always available. This may be due to the scarcity of organs or machines, the age of the person, either too old or too young, the person may be in an area where this is not available, or the person may be in such poor nutritional condition that they cannot tolerate the stress of surgery.

Gary had chronic kidney problems. His diseased kidneys were probably due to the diabetes that he suffered from for years. When I talked with him, he was in the hospital for dialysis again. He was completely blind in one eye and was rapidly losing sight in the remaining eye. Despite the condition of his body, Gary was a well person. He understood that his kidneys would completely fail some day and because of the diabetes he was not a candidate for a transplant. He enjoyed each day that he had. When the nurse would come into the room to perform some treatment on his one good eye he would patiently explain how the procedure worked best for him. He told me that it was important for him to know honestly what was happening to his body. He wanted to know everything that his physician could tell him about what to expect. He further stated that a person in his condition needed someone to talk to about his fears and concerns. He felt that this person could be anywhere as long as they were available by telephone. He needed this person to be one that he chose and one who was accessible to him for the duration of his disease. The person that he had chosen lived in Canada and their visits were primarily telephone visits.

It is important to realize that the kidneys do not work in a vacuum. They affect and are affected by other organ systems. The respiratory system and circulatory system are two of these systems. We have already discussed the circulatory system; next the respiratory system will be discussed.

The Respiratory System

The ability to breathe is absolutely necessary for life. Day by day and night after night we breathe continuously and rhythmically without paying any attention to this necessary, life- sustaining activity.

Overview of the Anatomy and Physiology of the Respiratory System.

The function of the respiratory system is for the exchange of gases. We take in oxygen, which is vital in constant supply for life to continue, and we breathe out carbon dioxide, a waste product of normal metabolism.

The relaxed adult breathes in and out 10 to 14 times per minute. The time from the beginning of one breath to the beginning of the next breath is about four to six seconds. Actually, you breathe in and out and then there is a short pause before the next breath begins. The resting adult with normal lung capacity will take in 9 to 12 pints of air each minute. With vigorous activity this can multiply by fifteen to twenty times. The panting adult will then be taking in as much as 20 gallons of air each minute. This is necessary because the resting adult has very little reserve of oxygen. So it only takes about twenty seconds of hard work to use up all the reserve oxygen in the lungs.

The respiratory system is divided into the upper and lower respiratory tracts. The upper respiratory tract consists of the nose, mouth, pharynx and larynx. The function of this tube-like structure is to warm and moisten the air that in inhaled. It also leads the air to the lower respiratory tract. The larynx contains the voice box; it is the air moving across this structure that allows us to talk.

The lower respiratory tract consists of the trachea, bronchi and lungs. The trachea, sometimes referred to as the windpipe, is simply a passageway. At the lower end of the trachea the pipe divides in half, forming the two bronchi. The bronchial tubes go to the right and the left and enter the lungs where they branch into smaller and smaller tubes called bronchioles. It looks much like a tree with the limbs dividing into more and more branches. In the lungs at the end of the bronchioles there are balloon-like structures called alveoli. The alveoli cluster like a bunch of grapes.

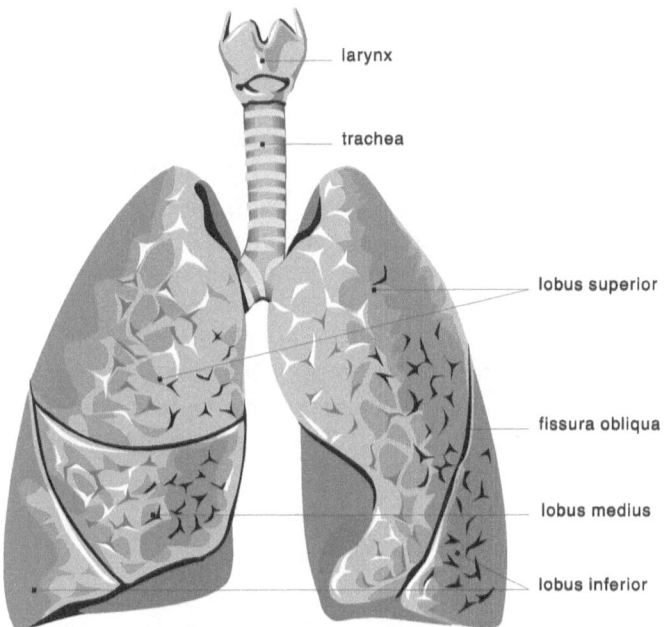

Figure 6: The Lungs

The lungs are formed into lobes. There are three lobes on the right lung and two lobes on the left lung. The reason the left lung has only two lobes is to leave space for the heart. When a person inhales, the alveoli inflate with air and when the person exhales the alveoli collapse like a balloon. There are about 300 million alveoli in the two lungs. It is in the alveoli that the gas exchange takes place. The vessels that enter the lungs branch into very small vessels so that the blood passes through cell by cell. As the red cells pass the alveoli the oxygen from the lung passes into the blood and the carbon dioxide from the blood passes into the alveoli.

Normally gas exchange occurs in half the time that is allowed for it. The blood is exposed to the alveoli for about 0.8 seconds in a resting adult.

The blood is saturated with oxygen in 0.4 seconds. Carbon dioxide exchange takes place 20 times faster than that. This gas exchange is dependent on proper pressure in both the lungs and the blood vessels, and normal ì alveolar structure. The blood is then pumped back into the heart and the carbon dioxide is thrown out of the body in exhaled air. The cycle goes on every minute of our lives, the rhythm being controlled by the respiratory center in the brain. Damage to the brain either due to injury or disease can interfere with the normal breathing patterns. They may become slow or rapid, shallow or deep.

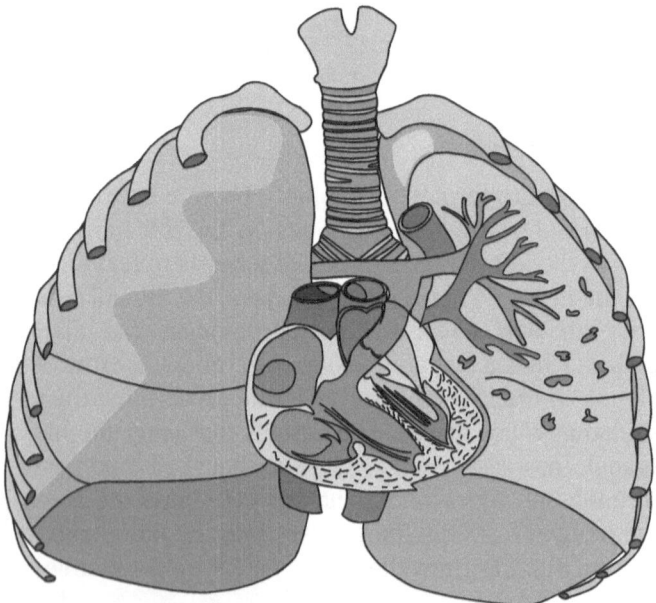

Figure 7: Chest Cavity

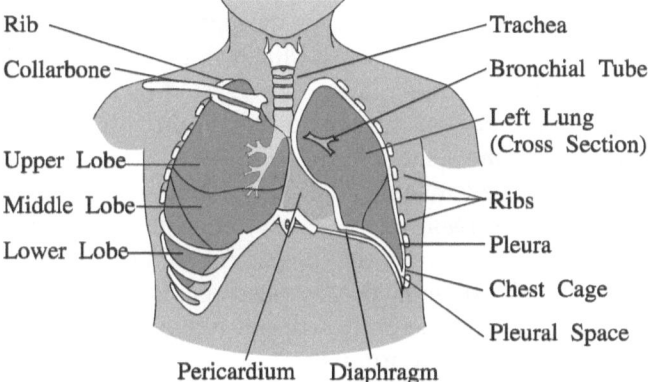
Figure 8: The Chest with Lungs Visible

What Happens To this System During the Dying Process

Although breathing is a very unconscious activity in a normal, healthy person, in the dying process breathing can change in several ways. If the primary disease is a respiratory problem the breathing patterns will have been different than normal for some time. A person with emphysema has difficulty exhaling because of the damage to the alveoli, therefore the breathing pattern will appear labored with very little activity long before the final dying process begins.

In the final stages of dying the person's breathing may become very erratic. It may be rapid and shallow or it may be slow and very deep. The two patterns may alternate over the period of an hour. Neither provides for sufficient exchange of oxygen in the lungs. As the breathing becomes inadequate for normal life you may notice a blueness around the lips and fingernail beds.

This is because not enough oxygen is being taken in to saturate the blood as it moves through the lungs. The eye lids may also take on a bluish tint. The level of consciousness may also decrease because of insufficient oxygen supply to the brain. Marathon runners at the end of the run will not process information adequately, because their overworked muscles are screaming for every molecule of oxygen that can be taken in by the lungs. As the body returns to normal the thought process also recovers, but with the dying person the body will not move towards that former level of equilibrium.

Certain characteristic breathing patterns are found in the dying person. Cheyne-Stokes ì is one of these. This form of respiration will occur within 24 hours of death. It is characterized by respirations that gradually increase in rate and depth until it reaches a peak. Then it gradually decreases in rate and depth until there is a pause in respiration. This is an indication that the respiratory center in the brain is not functioning normally. This may be due to disease, trauma or the dying process.

Another pattern of breathing is an exaggerated inspiration. This is like a person gasping for breath. This is called "air Hunger." As the person exhales there is be an audible sign. Biot's respiration is another pattern that may be observed. This occurs when respirations are rapid and deep followed by a pause.

A person suffering with lung disease will have an increase of secretions. It is normal to have some secretions in healthy tissue to keep it lubricated, but in diseased tissue as in the common cold there is an increased production of secretions. The accumulation of fluids may be great enough and uncomfortable enough that the secretions will need to be removed by suctioning. This procedure is very distressing to the person being suctioned. Early in the process the person will be able to cough the secretions out of the airway without help, but as the energy level decreases and sensations lessen the person could choke on their own secretions. Suctioning may be considered a comfort measure at this time. Suctioning is a very uncomfortable and distressing procedure in which a tube is pushed into the airway. The person has a definite feeling of not being able to breath. If this procedure is not done quickly and properly the person's natural instinct is to push the intruder away.

Lloyd was dying from lung cancer. The family had been alerted that death was a matter of hours away. The family took turns keeping vigil at the bedside. During the night secretions continued to build up at an increasing rate. Lloyd's son watched as the nurses repeatedly subjected his father to the trauma of secretion removal. As dawn was breaking Lloyd was once again being suctioned. His son noticed large tears begin to flow from his father's eyes. At this point the son said: "He has had enough. Leave him alone. Do not do that again." The nursing staff argued, but the son was adamant. When family members came to visit later that morning they could hear Lloyd's breathing when they stepped off the elevator. The family approved of the decision to allow Lloyd some peace. He died that morning without further stress of the suctioning tube.

The Living End

The cessation of breathing is a sign of death but there are problems with this as a single criteria. In ancient times it was believed that this was the only sign of life. The people around the dying held a feather or mirror before the nose to determine if the person was still breathing. When there was no movement of the feather or moisture on the mirror the person was declared dead. Today we know that this method of determining death can be inaccurate. The breathing may be very slow. The rate could be as low as four to five breaths per minute during the last few hours of life. As breathing becomes this slow the lack of oxygen affects other systems, since a steady supply of oxygen is essential for life. If the breathing is the first function to cease, the heart may continue for a few beats. After all vital functions have stopped for five to ten minutes there may be one final sigh. This is the final expiration from the lungs. This happens often in sudden death. It has sometimes caused uninformed observers to wonder if the person is truly dead. It is a startling event to witness if you are not prepared for it.

Mabel was in her barn when she had a heart attack. When she failed to return to the house her husband went to search for her. He found her lying in the barn, unresponsive. He called the rural volunteer ambulance. When the crew arrived they began CPR. After ten minutes there was still no response. The paramedic arrived and investigated the events in relation to probable time that Mabel had been without breathing.

The time that elapsed between collapse and CPR was at least a half hour and Mabel was well into her sixties with a history of heart disease. The paramedic knew that the chances of resuscitation were almost zero. She instructed the crew to discontinue CPR. Several seconds later Mabel gave out the final sigh. The ambulance crew observed this and then looked at the paramedic, questioning her judgment to discontinue CPR. When she explained they were satisfied.

Diseases of the Respiratory System

One of the most common diseases of the respiratory system is COPD. This stands for chronic obstructive pulmonary (lung) disease. It is an umbrella term which includes emphysema, chronic bronchitis, asthma, and cystic fibrosis. These diseases appear to be on the increase, probably because they are caused by irritating agents such as air pollution, smoke, industrial fumes, pollens, organic dusts, aging and harmful drugs and chemicals. All forms of COPD cause narrowing of the airway to and from the lungs. This narrowing traps air in the lungs and prevents normal gas exchange. The exact way that this happens varies with each disease.

Chronic bronchitis is a persistent irritation of the tissues in the bronchi and bronchioles. It is most often caused by cigarette smoke or air pollution. The irritation causes an increase in the production of mucus. This prevents normal air flow and gas exchange because air is not getting into and out of the alveoli. As the disease progresses, more alveoli are inadequately supplied with air causing the person to have a slight blue tint to the skin. Emphysema may develop after many years of chronic bronchitis

Emphysema is a degenerative disease of the lungs that causes the alveoli cluster to lose its ability to collapse after being inflated with air. It becomes one big sac instead of being a cluster. Air is trapped in the sack and there is less gas exchange area between the small blood vessels and the alveoli. The trapped air can only be removed from the lungs by forcefully exhaling, using not only the normal muscles of breathing, but also the muscles in the neck and abdomen. As the disease progresses the person will have chronic increase of carbon dioxide in the blood. The body can adjust to this, but it makes the use of concentrated oxygen in emergencies a problem. Increasing the saturation of oxygen in the blood can cause the respiratory center of the brain to slow respirations dangerously low. Ultimately the ì air sacs become so inadequate that normal activity is more and more ì difficult because the intake of air cannot keep up with the increase in demand. When this happens the heart will attempt to help by beating more forcefully and rapidly thus moving more blood through the lungs ì to soak up more oxygen. Eventually, with this increased activity of the heart muscle, the heart will enlarge and function less effectively. We ì then see congestive heart failure and all its complications.

Cheryl had been a smoker for many years. In her forties she was diagnosed as having emphysema. Her physician encouraged her to stop smoking, but Cheryl was stubborn and refused to follow his advice. By the time she was fifty Cheryl was an invalid. She could no longer do routine activities without becoming short of breath. Still she refused to give up smoking. Her physician realized with despair that there was little he could do for her as long as she continued to damage her lungs with the tar and nicotine of cigarette smoke.

Cheryl was losing weight and her disease continued to progress. The day came when she needed continuous oxygen to survive. Even then she would turn off the flow of oxygen for her cigarette. Then, wheezing and coughing, she resumed the oxygen, using her limited energy to recover from the smoke. By this time all who cared for her gave up trying to convince her that smoking was killing her. Finally, after years of fighting her disease, she quit smoking. Her lungs were so badly damaged that there was no hope for her recovery, but at least now she could use her diminished supply of energy to do her daily hygiene and feed herself. It had been many years since she had been able to do more than that. Several years after she quit smoking Cheryl's overworked heart and lungs finally gave out.

When the bronchi go into spasm the condition is known as asthma. It can be caused by infection, irritants, psychological stress, exercise or drugs. There is an increase in the production of mucus and plugs of this mucus obstruct the small airways making air exchange even more difficult and causing a wheezing sound on expiration. Usually asthma is treatable, but prolonged broncho-spasms can cause permanent narrowing of the airway. This leads to a disease process much like emphysema.

Cystic fibrosis is characterized by very thick mucus secretions. This results in obstruction of the alveoli in the lungs as well as the ducts in the liver and pancreas. When the person inhales, the air flows in normally, but then the airway collapses during exhalation trapping air in the lungs. The mucus that is then trapped causes infection, which produces more mucus that causes more obstruction. As the cycle continues the normal lung tissue is destroyed and normal gas exchange is impossible.

Pneumonia is an inflammation of the lungs. It can be caused by bacteria, virus, or aspirating foreign matter such as gastric juices, water, or hydrocarbons. The inflammation may involve alveoli, part of a lobe, the entire lobe or several lobes, as in double pneumonia. The organism or irritating agents enters the lung and causes inflammation. The affected area becomes swollen and pus-like fluid collects, interfering with normal gas exchange. The majority of pneumonias involve the lower part of the lungs and usually only one lobe is affected. In the upright person most gas exchange occurs in the lower part of the lung which is why most pneumonias occur there because there is greater exposure to the organism or irritating agents. This greater gas exchange in the lower lung also explains why there is more breathing difficulty when the pneumonia is located in the lower lung than when it occurs in the upper lobes.

A pneumonia may develop when a person is allowed to stay in one position for extended periods of time. This is one reason that unconscious, semi-conscious, debilitated, or anesthetized persons are turned every two hours. Pneumonia develops because there is not sufficient air exchange in the alveoli resulting in fluid accumulating in the air sacs. This stagnate fluid will cause the tissue to become raw and irritated. As air is breathed in containing the usual organism that would normally not affect healthy tissue the germs settle onto the red, swollen, warm area causing inflammation and pneumonia.

The Living End

Cancer of the lung is one of the leading causes of death in America. There is no question that it is directly linked to cigarette smoking. There are several kinds of cancer that affect the lung tissue. Some are very rapid growing and some are slower to develop, but all cancers cells reproduce more rapidly than normal tissue. Like uninvited guests the cancer cells crowd out the normal tissue and use up the nutrients intended for healthy cells. Cancer can be present anywhere along the respiratory tract, but it is more common in the lungs. It is easy to understand that as the healthy cells of the lungs are replaced by unhealthy cancer cells normal gas exchange will no longer be possible. As the cancer growth continues to increase and more and more lung tissue is squeezed out the oxygen in the body becomes to low to sustain life.

Jim had lung cancer. He had been a smoker for many years. He was in his mid forties, but his disease was killing him. He started smoking long before we really knew the connection between cigarette smoking and cancer of the lungs. Many nights he would wake up struggling for breath, begging for help. There was so little that could be done for him except comfort him and let him know that he was not alone. The cancer was replacing his normal lung tissue and we could only give concentrated oxygen so that what little lung tissue he had could put more oxygen into the blood. The day arrived when the oxygen level in his blood became so low that he mercifully lost consciousness and within twenty hours later he was dead. The saddest part of this situation was that when he went into the hospital he asked his wife and physician not to tell him about his condition and whether he would get well. His poor wife never had the comfort of being able to tell him goodbye.

A roaming blood clot can lodge anywhere and the lungs are no exception. These clots most often form in the legs. If they break lose they will travel through the blood vessels until they reach one that is small enough for it to lodge. Once the clot is stuck in a blood vessel in the lungs it will either stop or greatly decrease the flow of blood to that part of the lungs. This can cause pain and shortness of breath. The pain is caused by a lack of blood supply to the area. The shortness of breath is due to the inactivity of the part that is not receiving blood. Depending on the size of the area affected it can be an emergency or of little consequence.

Pulmonary edema occurs when fluid backs up into the tissue of the lungs. This is usually caused by heart disease that was covered in the chapter on that topic. When there is fluid in the lungs normal gas exchange does not occur. The person will breath with a wheezing sound. As the whole body slows activity during the dying process fluid often builds up in the tissue of the lungs. This is especially true if the person is receiving intravenous fluids. This lack of the body's ability to handle fluids lasts less than a week if the normal dying process is allowed to happen without interference.

There are many other diseases affecting the lungs. These are the disorders that will most often be encountered. As in most organ systems the disease process may be different, but the needs of the person as they endure the malady affecting them will be very similar. If the respiratory system is involved then getting enough oxygen to the cells of the body to maintain normal activity will be a dilemma.

The Nervous System

The brain, spinal cord and the nerves serve as our communication with the outside world and with our internal world. The brain controls what goes on in the rest of the body. In a normal adult, there is nothing that can happen to the body that the brain does not know about and have some control over. The brain can be compared to a super computer. Just as we program the computer, we program our brains. We decide what kind of an attitude to have about things; we react to situations according to our past experiences; and we learn to drive or do other skills through practice. Thus we program our brains. There are functions that the brain cannot do as rapidly as the computer can, but the brain is capable of far more complicated activities than the computer. After all, the computer is the result of the human brain. It is estimated that no one uses all of the potential that the brain has. This is what makes it possible to retrain people after part of the brain has been damaged.

In order to function properly, the brain must have a continuous supply of oxygen. It also needs glucose and cholesterol to work normally. The brain is so complicated that even though there has been a tremendous amount of research on the activity of the organ, we still have much to learn.

There is a new science called psychoneuroimmunology which studies how the brain affects the immune system. It is concerned with the ability of a person to have some control over the diseases that impact them. These are exciting times in brain research.

Overview of the Anatomy and Physiology of the Nervous System

The nervous system consists of the brain, the spinal cord, and the nerves. The brain is the master controller. Messages are sent to the brain for interpretation and instructions.

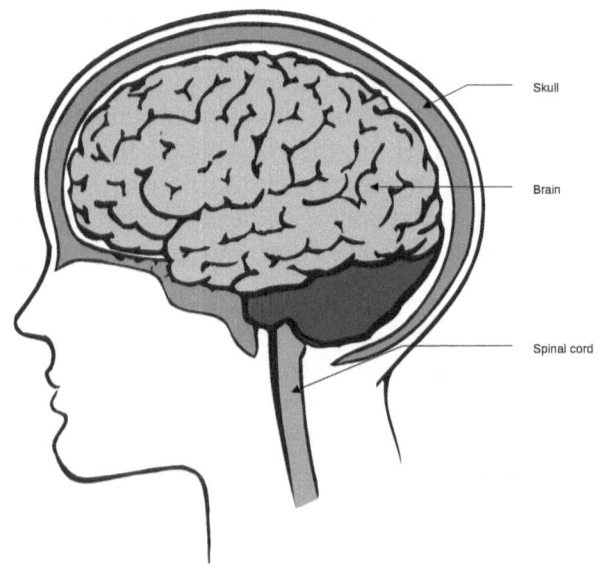

Figure 9: The brain Inside the Scull

The adult brain weighs about three pounds. It is a soft lump of over fourteen million cells. It is so limp that if

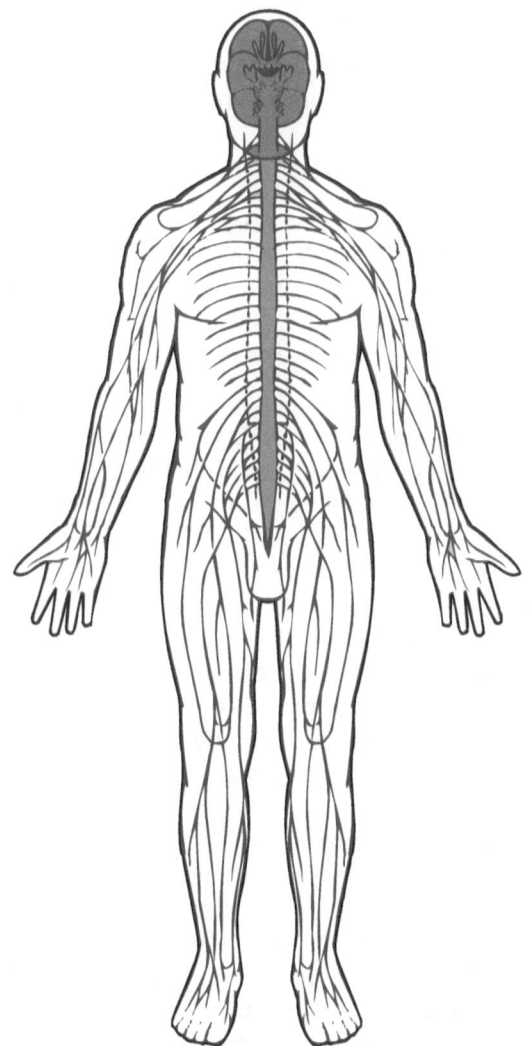

Figure 10: The Nervous System

it is placed on a table without the firm support of its covering it will spread out like spilled milk. It is like a very large piece of paper that has been crunched up into many convolutions. The size of the brain has very little to do with ability and intelligence; although we know that to be accused of having a bird brain is not a compliment.

The brain is protected by the bony structure of the skull. An infant's brain is proportionately larger than the adult brain. It grows slower than the rest of the body after birth and reaches its final size at approximately nine years of age. At birth the skull has separations between the bones that allow for this growth.

There are four parts to the brain (Figure 11). The cerebrum is located in the top of the head. This is the site of the highest intellectual function. It is this part that the lower animals do not have. The mid-brain lies between the cerebrum and the cerebellum. It contains the thalamus and hypothalamus, but mostly it is a passage between two very important structures. The cerebellum lies in the back of the head. The function of this part of the brain is to control the skeletal muscles. It coordinates the movement of groups of muscles, maintains equilibrium, and helps control posture. It functions on the unconscious level to ensure that our movements are smooth, efficient, and effective. When fly buzzes around your head, without thinking you accurately swat it away from you. The brain stem lies below the cerebellum and connects the brain to the spinal cord. This structure performs sensory, motor, and reflex functions. Some of these are vital functions necessary for survival. It controls the reflex for heart action, blood vessel diameter, and respiration. A severe blow to this part of the head can cause instant death. It is also the center for non- vital reflexes such as sneezing, vomiting, coughing, and swallowing. The nerve impulses that do not require reflex action continue on to the higher brain. The nerves coming from the spinal cord cross in this structure so that messages from the right side of the body go to the left side of the brain. That is why injury to the left side of the brain will cause motion and sensory problems on the right side of the body.

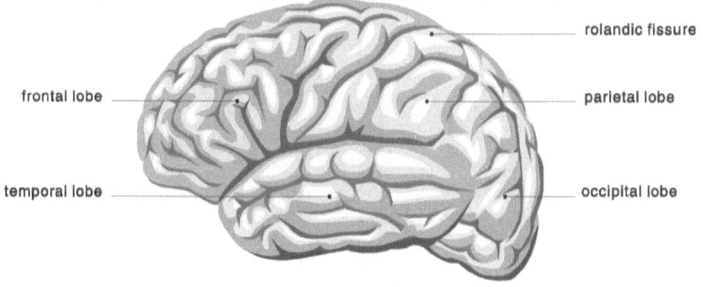

Figure 11: The Brain

The spinal cord lies within the bony structure of the back bone, or vertebrae. It is about seventeen inches long in the adult. It is oval-shaped and tapers slightly from its beginning at the brain stem to the end slightly below the waist. All along the way nerves branch off the spinal cord. The function of the spinal cord is to pass messages from the outside world and inside world to and from the brain. It is also responsible for some reflex actions. If you touch your hand to a very hot stove, the reflex from the spinal cord will pull your hand away from danger long before the message reaches the brain that the stove is hot.

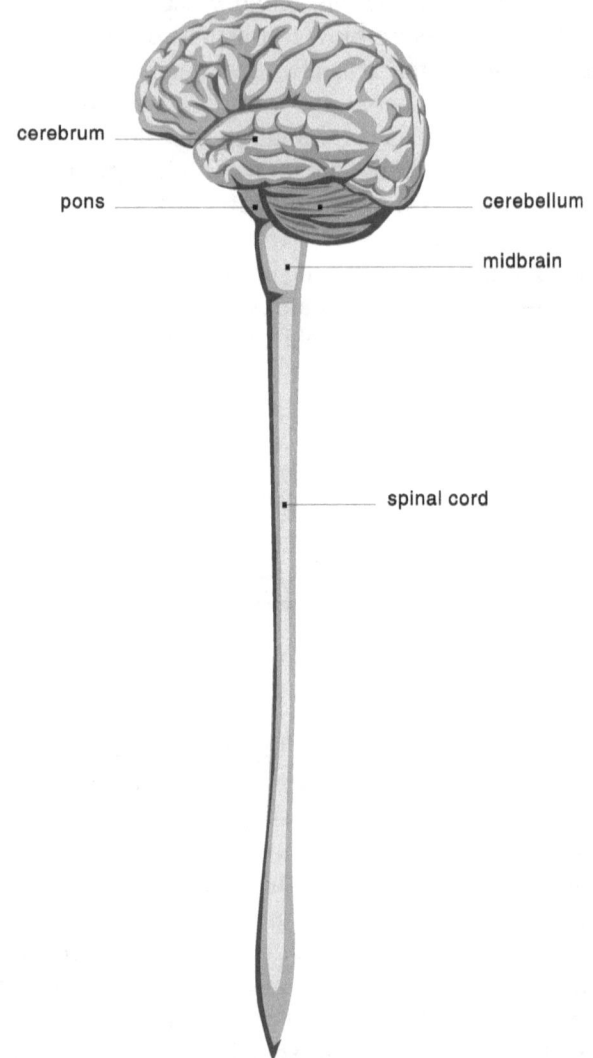

Figure 12: Brain with Spinal Cord

The Living End

The brain and spinal cord are covered by a membrane called meninges. There are three layers to this covering. The outer layer is a tough fibrous tissue called the dura mater (this is Latin meaning tough mother). The middle layer is a cobwebby, delicate material called the arachnoid membrane. The inner layer, called the pia mater, sticks to the surface of the brain and spinal cord; it is transparent and contains blood vessels. There is a microscopic space between each of these layers. There is fluid in the space known as the subarachnoid space which is the space between the arachnoid and the pia mater. The purpose of this fluid is to cushion the brain and spinal cord. If this fluid was absent, than every time you moved your head abruptly your brain would smash against the rough bony structure of your skull. This would cause the brain to bruise and you would have what is known as a concussion. None of us would survive childhood if our brains were not cushioned this way.

Nerves are all over your body (Figure 10: The Nervous System). There are nerves that sense hot, nerves that sense cold, nerves that sense pain, nerves that sense pressure, nerves that sense tension, nerves that sense stretching. The nerves are specialized and all sensation is not equally distributed. You will notice that when you are out in very cold weather you feel the coldness on your face and hands, but you are surprised when you touch your thigh with your hand to feel the coldness there also. You can tolerate a pin prick on your back with less pain than on your lip. The heart muscle has no pain receptors. The pain from a heart attack comes from surrounding tissue.

How the Dying Process Affects the System

Some very important changes occur in this system during the dying process. If the brain is the primary site of disease, the events will be different than when other areas of the body are the primary cause of death.

Let us first consider the patient with disease of some part of the body other than the brain. The level of consciousness will decrease so that the person will sometimes be alert and well oriented as to time, place and person. They will recognize everyone that they have known in the past and will be able to carry on a normal conversation. There will be other times when they will seem preoccupied with their own thoughts. They may not recognize family and friends and they will show little interest in what is going on around them. This may occur from time to time during the course of the illness, but it will become more pronounced during the last week or two. At first, the times of alertness will be longer than the times of detachment. As death approaches, the periods of detachment will increase. For many people, the last day or more will be spent in coma.

The event that can be very confusing to the family concerns the sudden period when the dying person is alert and lucid after several days of near coma or even complete coma. This event usually occurs a day before death and is caused by the erratic release of adrenalin during the final stages of dying. It seems that the dying person needs this final chance to say "goodbye." If the family does not understand this occurrence, they will revive the hope that the dying person will recover after all.

Although the person may not be responding much to outside stimuli, the sense of touch is enhanced. Think of a time when you were half asleep or anesthetized. Remember how irritating it was to be stroked or moved. The dying person feels this same irritation. This explains why the person will throw off the covers and attempt to be free from intravenous needles and tubing, oxygen tubing, tubing leading into the stomach, and any other equipment that is touching the sensitive skin.

Holding the dying person's hand or placing your hand gently on an arm is comforting. It allows the person to know that a caring individual is there. It is a soothing non-verbal way to share with the dying person. This activity should be encouraged, but patting, stroking, and moving the dying person around should be avoided as much as possible.

Good nursing procedure includes making sure that a bedridden person is moved every two hours. When the person does not or is unable to do this unaided, then they are passively moved by the nursing staff. There are many good reasons for this procedure-- to help prevent static pneumonia and pressure sores, to smooth wrinkles from bed linens, and to clean the body. When caring for a dying person these reasons lose validity. Most of the dying express their desire to be left in peace by moaning and "fighting back." This "fighting back" involves pushing caretakers away, waving arms and legs in the air, shaking the head from side to side, or many other non-verbal negative messages. This makes it difficult for the caretaker to succeed in moving the dying person. It is like a battle with each participant intent on victory. Unfortunately,

The Living End

ì it is the caretakers who usually get their way. They proceed to their next assignment with a sense of satisfaction while the person they are presumed to be helping once again has lost control. We need to pay attention to these messages from the dying people. They are trying to tell us that they want to be handled as little as possible, and then when they are moved-- **"please handle with care."**

There is a phenomenon known as "picking of bed covers." This is sometimes observed a day or two before death. The person seems to be attempting to pick up tiny objects from off their covers. It may be that they are trying to remove the covers from their body because the increased sensitivity of their skin is causing them to be irritating.

Even when a person appears to be unconscious, the hearing is still intact. The hearing is the last sense to function. We learn of many people who can report exactly what was said in their presence when they were unconscious.

Henry was in kidney failure. He was brought to the emergency department unresponsive. The medical staff was discussing his condition within his hearing. They were trying to decide how aggressively to treat him. Henry could hear and process everything that was being said. He struggled in his mind to communicate the message: "Please don't let me die. Do what you need to so I can live." Henry lived to tell that story.

Knowing this about Henry, you should talk to the unconscious in a normal way. Even when you are not sure that the person is processing what you have to say, continue to communicate. Many, many years ago in my student nurse days, I cared for a young man who was the victim of a serious automobile accident. In those days there were no intensive care units so this dying person was assigned to my area. It was tragic to watch the mother stand by his bedside, holding his hand and saying over and over: "Please don't die. Please don't die." The young man struggled to speak with his mother, but his head and face injuries were too great. His grieving mother watched him die. Now after many years experience, I know his dying would have been more peaceful for everyone if his mother could have recognized that he could not live. She would have been able to release him as Elizabeth's husband was able to do.

In the dying person, the temperature may begin to rise. This is misunderstood by many people. There is a temperature control center in the brain. This allows the body to respond with a fever to fight infections. In the dying person this center may malfunction causing the temperature to either rise or fall. Normally we attempt to lower a high temperature to prevent the destruction of brain tissue. However, when a person is dying, there is no reason to subject them to the discomfort of cooling methods. It may be argued that a fever is uncomfortable, because when healthy people run fevers they feel sick. That is because we are trying to carry on our normal daily activities. The fever in itself is not uncomfortable. The dying person does not feel troubled ì by the fever. The methods for lowering the temperature, however, make the person uneasy and usually are not very effective. The temperature may come down for a short period of time, but it will rise again.

One method used for lowering temperatures in the dying person is a cooling blanket. It is like a large ice pack and it is heavier than a blanket. It is usually placed over the person. The idea is to lower the skin temperature and this will ultimately lower the internal temperature. Since you already know that the circulation of the dying person is slowing down, you understand why this has little effect. Many people who have had this blanket used on them have told how distressing it is.

I remember a young boy who had a non-life threatening infection. His temperature was very high and anti-pyretics were not being effective. His physician ordered that this cooling blanket be used when his temperature was very high. After it was used his temperature lowered, but it elevated again. This young boy cried and pleaded with us not to subject him to this unpleasant procedure. It was necessary for him and we successfully explained that to him.

As the person's body continues to decline, other systems controlled by the nervous system are affected. The person loses control of urine and feces. Sometimes this will begin as much as a week or two before death. At other times, it will occur simultaneously with death.

We learn bladder and bowel control as small children. It is reasonable that when someone has lost conscious control of other body parts that the bladder and bowel control would also be lost. This is very distressing to family members. It is important to keep these events in perspective. It is a normal occurrence and should not be a cause for concern or embarrassment.

When the brain is the primary site of disease, unconsciousness may occur weeks before death comes. Before the person loses responsiveness, they may have periods when they are confused, irrational, unreasonable, belligerent, and quarrelsome. This is a difficult time, but you must remember it is the disease causing this unusual behavior.

The person may become very combative and violent. It may be serious enough that the lives of the person, staff and family are in danger. At this time, it will be necessary to sedate the person. It is really the only humane thing to do. The person is not choosing to act this way. Their disease is interfering with rational behavior. For their own dignity and the safety of all, sedation is the best course of action.

Diseases of the Nervous System

A cardiovascular accident (CVA), or stroke, is the leading cause of death in diseases of the nervous system. It has been said that if nothing else kills you, a stroke will.

A stroke is an interruption in the normal flow of blood to the brain. The most common causes are thrombus, embolus or hemorrhage. The severity of the stroke will depend on where in the brain the accident occurs. If it affects a large vital area, the stroke may be immediately fatal. If a small vessel flow is involved, the person will experience what is called a TIA or transient ischemia attack.

A stroke due to thrombus is the most common type of CVA. The inside area of arteries becomes smaller in aging people because of hardening of these arteries. The opening in the vessel becomes smaller and smaller until eventually no blood can flow through the vessel. This can happen to any vessel thus stopping blood flow to the area past the occluded artery and producing a stroke. Hardening of the arteries or atherosclerosis is a normal consequence of living, but life style dictates how quickly this will become a problem. We know that those who eat healthy, exercise, and are well mentally, spiritually and emotionally are less prone to experience the effects of atherosclerosis early in life.

An embolism may occur at anytime in life. It is a foreign particle that floats in the vessels until it lodges in a vessel that is smaller than the particle. These particles may be blood clots or fat molecule that arise from some other part of the body. One of the dangers of any surgery is the possibility of these types of blood clots. A fat embolus is possible after fracturing a bone. In the vast majority of surgeries and fractures these emboli do not happen, but the potential is there.

Hemorrhages in the brain can also develop at any age. They may be due to a genetic defect, injury to the head, or damage to the vessels due to chronic high blood pressure. In these cases, the vessel is ruptured allowing blood to leak into the surrounding brain tissue. As the blood accumulates, further damage is done because the tissue and vessels are being squeezed and no blood flow is getting through.

An aneurysm may be the cause of a brain hemorrhage. This is a ballooning out on the side of an artery because of a weakness in the wall of the vessel. This flaw in the artery may be genetic or due to trauma or aging. The weakness may not cause a problem until middle age when hardening of the arteries and high blood pressure cause an increase in turbulence and abnormal blood flow in the vessel. With the increase in pressure the vessel balloons out. The walls of the artery become thinner and thinner until ultimately they rupture. These weaknesses occur most often where vessels divide or branch off.

The term "brain tumor" strikes fear into the hearts of those who hear it. Because the brain is contained in the hard unyielding skull no swelling or abnormal growth can occur without serious damage to the brain tissue. Tumors may be benign or malignant. Either one must be removed or shrunk because there is no room for it. The good news is that brain cancers do not metastasize to other parts of the body. The bad news is that cancers in other parts of the body, like breast cancers, can metastasize to the brain.

There can be tumors on the spine. Many times these tumors arise from some other part of the body and then invade the spine. A tumor may be outside the spinal cord or inside the spinal cord. These tumors cause a lot of pain and disability.

Infections can be located anywhere in the brain or spinal cord. Meningitis ì is an infection of the lining of the brain and spinal cord. Acute meningitis can be due to either bacteria or virus. Even though we have antibiotics that are very effective in the treatment of many bacterial infections, people still die as the result of meningitis. I will always remember the two-year old child that I cared for years and years ago as a student nurse. Her diagnosis was bacterial meningitis. This little girl was the daughter of one of my teachers. The little girl was unconscious. Her disease was advanced enough that her little back was arched backwards so that she looked like the letter C. I spend hours standing at her bedside talking to her, singing to her, and praying that a miracle would happen and she would recover. She was such a beautiful child and I loved her. Even after I was moved to another nursing unit, I continued to visit this child. A miracle did not happen and I was sad when she died. Just a few days ago a young woman died from meningitis, so we haven't made much progress in treating that disease.

Subacute meningitis is caused by fungal infections, tuberculous or syphilis. The onset of this type is slower then the acute and lasts longer. It is also subject to relapses.

Any blow to the head can cause serious damage to the brain. The brain is so soft and the skull is hard. When the head is suddenly impacted, the brain smashes again the skull. This can cause bruising of the tissue or rupture of large vessel resulting in hemorrhage. A large bleed is life threatening and must be treated as an emergency.

There are several degenerative diseases of the nervous system. Multiple sclerosis is a chronic progressive disease which causes the degeneration of the covering of the nerves. It is marked by frequent reoccurrences and abatements. Myasthenia gravis has an unknown cause. It triggers an interference with the transmission of messages from the brain to the voluntary muscles.

This results in extreme muscle weakness. Ultimately there is an inability to speak, swallow, or maintain an open airway. With an inadequate airway, a respiratory emergency and death occurs. Muscular dystrophy is believed to be caused by a genetic defect. It results in progressive weakness and atrophy of the muscles. The person with this disease can look forward to being completely helpless.

The Digestive System

The year that my brother, Lou, was to celebrate his sixtieth birthday did not start out well for him. The pain in his lower back, that he had complained about in November, was continuing to bother him. When he had first experienced the pain, he had consulted a physician and the diagnosis was strained muscles. The second week in January, Lou developed abdominal pain and began vomiting. He thought he had picked up a "bug" so he endured his misery and thought it would clear-up in a day or so. His symptoms persisted. A week later, he was a very sick man and was admitted to the hospital. After the usual "tests" his physician decided that surgery was necessary because it was determined that he had an abdominal obstruction. In surgery, they found that this obstruction was a cancerous growth that involved not only his colon, but his kidneys and pelvic area. The pain that he had been experiencing in November was not back strain, but cancer. The outlook was bleak. My brother suffered through chemotherapy for several months. He died the middle of April after three months of real suffering. The one thing that he feared most was constant pain. He was spared this.

Overview of the Anatomy and Physiology of the Digestive System

The digestive system is anatomically very simple and physiologically very complex. Structurally, it is just a tube that starts with the mouth and ends with the rectum. There are bulges and narrowings along the way, but it is a continuous hollow tube. What happens inside that tube is complicated, baffling, marvelous, magical and absolutely essential to life and health.

The mouth receives food. Saliva is mixed with the food as it is chewed and broken into small enough particles to be swallowed. The esophagus is the hallway between the mouth and the stomach. Very little digestion occurs in the stomach. It is basically a pouch that holds the food before it is passed into the intestines. The stomach expands with food and as the contents leave the stomach, this pouch contracts. The mystifying part of the stomach is that it secretes hydrochloric acid that breaks down meat into usable substance for the intestines and yet it does not digest the stomach itself. The hydrochloric acid is so strong that it could burn a hole in the carpet. A healthy person has no problem with burns of the stomach. We do know that this does become a problem for those with chronic stress.

The tube narrows for the small intestines. The small intestines measure about an inch in diameter and are twenty feet long. They coil and loop to fill the abdominal cavity. The greater part of digestion occurs in the small intestines. They complete the breakdown of food into protein, carbohydrates and fats and then these nutrients are absorbed into the blood. These essential end-products of digestion are then distributed to all the cells of the body.

The last part of the digestive tube is the large intestines. It measures about two and a half inches in diameter and is approximately five feet long. The rectum is the last seven inches of the large intestines. The main function of the large intestines is to absorb water from the material that is passing through and then to eliminate the waste produces of digestion.

There is a motion called peristalsis that moves the contents of the digestive system along. Ordinarily, this motion is smooth and gentle. The material moves along at a rate that allows for proper metabolism. When the rate is increased a person experiences

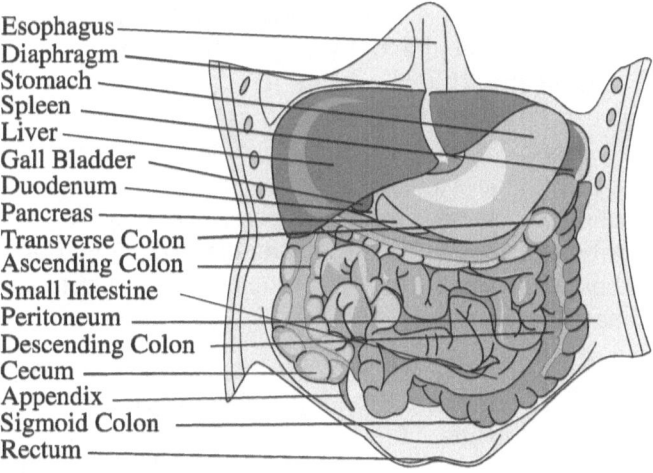

Figure 13: Abdominal Digestive Organs

diarrhea; but if the rate slows very much an obstruction may form or the person may simply encounter constipation. Acute stress may initially cause a slowing of peristalsis, but then the rate will increase past normal causing diarrhea. Chronic stress sometimes triggers persistent diarrhea. This may ultimately become a serious problem.

Several accessory organs are essential for normal digestion. The pancreas is a small gland that measures six to nine inches long and lies just below the stomach. This gland secretes several enzymes that are needed for metabolism. Among these is insulin, which is decreased or lacking in diabetics. Insulin is necessary for the metabolism of carbohydrates.

The liver is the largest gland in the body. It lies just below the diaphragm and to the right. It is shaped like a triangle with the straight sides just under the diaphragm and down the right side extending from the fourth rib to the last rib. The slanted side goes from the tenth rib on the right to just below and in the middle of the fifth rib on the left. The liver weighs between three and four pounds. This gland has many functions. The most important are: to detoxify substances that enter the body, such as drugs and alcohol; to secrete bile, which is needed for fat metabolism; to aid in the metabolism of protein and carbohydrates; and to store substances such as iron and some vitamins.

The gallbladder is well-known by many people as a source of pain and discomfort. This pear-shaped sac lies below the liver. It is only three to four inches long, but can hold about an ounce of bile. It's function is to store bile from the liver and then eject this bile into the stomach or small intestines as needed for digestion.

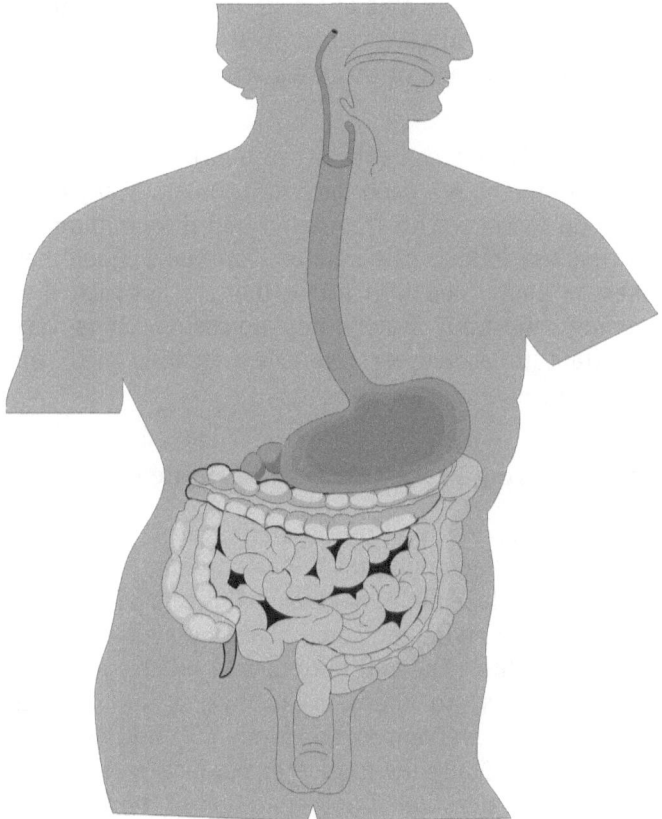

Figure 14: The Digestive System

Our appetites are controlled by the brain. Pleasing smells or a delicious looking food dish may trigger hunger. We also feel hungry at the times of day when we usually eat. This is because we are conditioned to eat at regular intervals. This is all regulated by the brain. If we couldn't consciously manage when we eat we would become out of control if we experienced hunger and were not able to satisfy the feeling. A baby will scream relentlessly when they feel hungry. No amount of reasoning or placating will satisfy their need for food.

We know that we can experience hunger, which is not related to the body's need for nourishment. Many of us use food to cope with frustration and disappointment. We also use food to celebrate and entertain. Food then takes on many meanings for us that are not related to keeping the body functioning normally. It is very important to remember this when dealing with the dying person.

How the Dying Process Affects this System

Alterations in the digestive system may occur earlier than many other symptoms. It is common for people who are ill to lose their appetites and this is particularly true with the dying person. There may be several reasons for this. The ability to taste food changes with many diseases, so there is a physical as well as psychological aversion to the foods that normally are favored. Physically the food does not taste as expected so the person questions the preparation of the food and they are disappointed that their favorite foods no longer give them the joy that they once did. This may all occur on the unconscious level, but it is happening. Think of the times when you have suffered from nausea. The smell of food was sickening, even your special food. The difference is that you knew that this condition was temporary and you would be back to normal soon. The dying person has no such assurance. This is disappointing and dismal at the very least.

The lose of appetite may be due to chemical changes in the body which stimulate appetite. This causes a general loss of interest in food. Since we associate wellness and health with an interest in food, many family members will attempt to tantalize the dying person as a method of assuring themselves that the person is not as near death as they fear. Many times the dying person will choke down food just to ease the suffering of the family. If the person does not want to eat, they should not be harassed. We should listen to the person and give them control of this last function, that of eating.

Harold was sent home to die. There was nothing more that the medical world could do for him. He was so happy because he wanted to be able to sit and look out over the farm that he loved and had worked for so many years. His wife was elated to have her husband home so that she could take care of him. After all, they had been together for over forty years and she didn't know how to NOT take care of him. She fixed all of his favorite foods and set the table as she had for many years. All was normal again. Poor Harold came to the table and smiling at his wife he sat down. He picked up his fork and transferred a bite to his mouth. He chewed and chewed, but he just couldn't swallow. He just couldn't eat. This caused so much pain, so much suffering for both of them. The wife flustered about and wanted to fix something different. The magic spell was broken. In despair the man left the table and, with tears streaming down her face, the wife cleared away the uneaten meal. If only she had been informed that small simple meals are better for dying people this tragedy would not have been. As it happened that was this man's last meal. The miserable widow was left to remember the last disastrous meal that she served her husband.

As the food intake decreases, the body will begin to use its own stored fat for energy to carry on normal functions. This will give the person a breath that smells like acetone; this is a normal by-product of burning or utilizing body fat. This can also be noted in a person who is on a strict weight reduction diet.

With the lower intake of food, the person will have less energy because of the diminished sugar consumption. The energy level of the cancer person is often lower than that of other people given the same nourishment level because the cancer continues to grow and use the nutrients even while the normal body tissue is deteriorating. This is the difficulty with cancer. It will grow at the expense of its host, just like a parasite.

With the total oral intake being decreased, fluids will also be taken in a lower quantity than is needed for a healthy body. The person will become slowly dehydrated. This will be impossible to detect at first without laboratory tests, but after a week the skin will begin to loss some of it's turgor. You will notice that when you pinch the skin it will stay in a peak longer than it will in a fully hydrated person. As time passes, this loss of turgor will increase. The amount of urine per day will decrease and it will look darker.

As dehydration increases the urine will be very concentrated and will appear very dark with an unpleasant odor. It is not unusual for the urine output to completely cease one or two days before death.

The tongue and mouth will become dry. It is a comfort measure to moisten these with damp compresses. An effort should be made to keep the mouth and tongue clean. They can become encrusted with dead tissue because the person will breath through the mouth.

At this time the medical staff will be tempted to recommend that IV fluids be initiated. Some view this dehydration as an isolated event that should be corrected instead of acknowledging it as a part of the total picture. Dehydration is not an enemy to the dying person. As dehydration progresses, the congestion in the lungs will lessen. Secretions ì that have been bothersome in the nose and throat will diminish.

It is reasonable to expect the glucose or sugar level in the blood to increase at this time. This has been observed in some people who have had blood work done at this point. An increase in the glucose now does not have the same significance that it has with a normal person. It is not unpleasant for the person and does not need to be treated. It is simply a normal event as the body chemistry progresses towards death. The important thing is to know that this may occur and it is not a reason for alarm.

During this time of decrease in oral intake, the activity of the intestines is slowing. This slowing will occur even if an attempt is made to artifically feed the person. There may be no stools for several days. There is simply no accumulation of material for stools and the normal activity of the intestinal tract is so diminished that there is no normal formation.

The circulation has also decreased to the intestines enough that the fluid in the large intestines is not being absorbed back into the blood vessels. In some people there may be a very liquid, foul smelling brown discharge from the rectum.

Mary was a dear little lady who had faithfully waited at her husband's bedside during the final days of his life. The staff knew that he was seriously ill, but they failed to adequately impress on her that her husband was dying. For several days before his death the husband had no stools and the wife was very concerned. She persistently asked the nursing staff to attend to what she perceived as a vital need-- a stool each day. When the her husband died, Mary was overcome with grief and continued to insist that if he had just had a stool he would not have died. This is incredibly sad and could have been avoided if someone had just explained to this lady what was happening to her husband. Then she could have been better prepared. She would have been able to say the things to her husband that she wanted to say before he died.

Diseases of the Digestive System

It is estimated that about 11 per cent of the population suffer from peptic ulcers. An ulcer is as an erosion of the normal tissue, causing a sore irritated area. Peptic ulcers occur in the wall of the stomach, pylorus (the sphincter between the stomach and the beginning of the small intestines), or the duodenum (the first part of the small intestines. The erosion of the tissue can affect the top layer, extend deep into the muscle tissue, or continue all the way through the wall into the surrounding area. The last condition is life threatening unless treated rapidly and aggressively. A hole in the wall of the stomach or small intestines allows the contents of these structures to leak into the abdominal cavity and a severe infection results. This is known as peritonitis. This ì infection progresses quickly and the person becomes very ill. They have acute pain and a very high fever. When ulcers are treated early and effectively this does not happen. The problem is that the treatment requires great discipline on the part of the person with an ulcer. If they ordinarily had this healthy lifestyle, the ulcer would have had less of a chance to develop.

Ulcerative colitis is an inflammation of the colon and rectum. This infection causes many small ulcers to form along this tissue. The exact cause of this condition is not known, but it is believed to be related to a lifestyle that is filled with stressful situations. This is a chronic disease and is complicated to treat. It has a high mortality rate. Because the disease is characterized by periods of exacerbations and remissions about 10 per cent of the people with this disease eventually develop cancer of the colon.

Tumors can occur anywhere along the digestive tract. A tumor may be cancerous, but it is not always. One of the most common causes of death from cancer is that of the colon (the large intestines). It is not absolutely known why cancer develops in the colon, but there is evidence that diet plays a big role in this. That certainly is logical since the function of the colon is to handle the by-produces of digestion.

Another disease that is chronic, but can become life threatening is diverticulosis. This occurs in 5 to 10 per cent of adults and usually develops over the age of 40. Diverticulosis is the presence of small sacs along the intestines. Those that appear in the large intestines are more likely to cause problems that those in the small intestines. The sacs may become inflamed and cause crampy pain, fever and nausea. This inflammation can lead to a perforation of the large intestines and peritonitis. Another emergency condition is created if the colon becomes obstructed because of the bulging sacs and inflammation. When the tube-like colon is closed off, its contents can no longer be emptied, but the intestines continue to produce materials from digestion. This causes a back-up in the colon much like a traffic jam. The person begins to vomit, has severe pain and becomes very ill. Surgery is usually indicated to remove the obstruction. If this is not done in timely fashion the colon will rupture and life-threatening peritonitis will result.

The list of diseases of the digestive system is not long. The number of people affected by this short list is very long. Many of us will go though life without experiencing a broken bone, pneumonia, or heart disease, but none of us will reach adulthood without having had at least one stomachache. While it may be embarrassing to have diarrhea, all of us have experienced it and can empathize with those suffering from an acute bout of the disease. This sets the digestive diseases apart from other illness. We can really relate to the person suffering abdominal pain.

Some Final Comments

There are some other ideas that do not fit in any of the other chapters. These are concepts that are useful to anyone concerned with the dying process. They ì deal mostly with honesty. Honesty on the part of the family as well as the medical profession. It is only fair to be honest.

There are times when the dying person is alert and lucid until the final seconds of life. It is difficult to completely grasp that the person is actually dying. You may be struck with the idea that the body is betraying the whole person in these situations. This illustrates that the essence of the person is still well even though the body has reached its limit. You will notice that these people exhibit the detachment that was discussed in the chapter on emotions. They are alert and able to communicate in a meaningful way, but they are not of this world.

It is important for the alert person to know about the progress of their disease. They are aware of the changes on the unconscious level, but they need the medical professionals and others around them to be completely honest and candid about their condition. This does not involve a morbid accounting of every detail. It means that questions, both verbal and non-verbal, should be answered factually. This may be the responsibility of the family if the physicians and nurses seem hesitant to do so.

Sometimes the dying person may state that they don't want to know the truth. This presents a dilemma for the family, because open dialogue about the person's future will be best for all of them. The dying person knows that their condition is terminal, but they may think it is best for the family to deny this reality until it happens. Sometimes the family may have a tradition of not openly discussing family matters. While this attitude should be respected, everyone will be able to handle the coming events with more peace if they can learn to share the experience.

The well-informed dying person and the family can cope with reality. It is difficult and painful to be left to struggle with what their imaginations present as the future. Armed with misinformation about the conceivable outcome for the dying person, all people concerned become more apprehensive ì unless they are thoroughly and honestly informed about the real situation. It is cruel and unjust to be told by busy, healthy people that: " everything is going to be all right" when the situation is obviously grave.

Michael was rushed to the hospital after suffering a severe heart attack. His family had a sense that he was not going to survive, but an emergency room personnel assured them that Michael was going to be fine and shooed them into the waiting room. There they discussed what the medical professional had told them and began to have hope that Michael would live. At that time the emergency personnel were frantic to bring life back to Michael. They failed. To assure the family that their husband and father was " going to be fine" was not appropriate and caused the family a lot of grief. For a long time afterwards they questioned the right of the hospital to misinform them.

The problem we face is that often the medical professional has trouble in dealing with death themselves. They may have never faced the death of someone close to them, so they cannot relate to the family in an empathic way. Sometimes they have not come to grips with the reality of their own mortality, so they shun those who are facing death almost as though they thought it was contagious. They intend to be compassionate and understanding, but they are fighting their own battle and therefore they appear unconcerned and callous. Forgive these people and find someone who can give you the support that you need.

An interesting phenomenon is that the dying people need to educate their own families about their disease and the ultimate outcome. The reason for this is that it helps the dying person with the reality of what is happening. When the dying person understands what is occurring and is able to talk about this to the family it helps everyone understand and share how the eventual death will affect the family. The subject of death is then removed from the area of the "unmentionable" to a point where it can be openly and freely discussed. Talking frankly helps the dying person through the final dying process. When the person knows he has been the educator for their family, he retains some control. This is very important to someone who has had to give up control over so many other areas.

Treating the dying person honestly will help the family adjust after death has occurred. They will have the comfort of knowing that they helped the one who died have a peaceful death. The dying person can help plan their own funeral. This benefits the family by not having to make final arrangements alone. In <u>A Severe Mercy</u>, Sheldon Vanauhen describes the peace he felt about his dead wife because they had planned her final tribute together. He knew he was doing it the way she wanted it done and he felt a closeness to her and an acceptance of the reality of her death.

The person who is facing death needs someone special to talk with. This someone does not need to be a professional counselor, but a confidante who is available anytime. They don't need to live in the same town as long as they are available by telephone.

In many hospice programs, the dying person is assigned a counselor or guide. This works well if there is good rapport between the two people. It would be better if the dying person was introduced to several possible confidantes and the one most affected could then choose the confidante they felt most comfortable with. It is often difficult for the dying person to talk freely with several people. That is why it is important to find that special person who will allow the dying person to share openly and freely.

The young person who is dying has special needs. They may never have seen a dead person except in the media. Perhaps they have not experienced the death of a family member. This situation will make the dying process even more frightening. They will want details about what will happen to them as they die and what other people will be experiencing. Someone who understands this need and can explain in detail will be beneficial to this young person.

Mary was in her early twenties, but she was dying. She asked to be taken to the room of another dying person so that they could share what was happening to them. She also wanted to see a dead body, because she had never seen one. It gave her peace when the dying process was explained to her and she was able to understand what would happen to her as she died.

In dealing with death we need to remember that every life is important. The way that each of us lives our life is unique. Each of us may die as uniquely as we have lived. There is not one right way to die. Emerson says it very well:

> "All things are engaged in writing their history. The plant, the pebble, goes attended by its shadow. The rolling rock leaves its scratches on the mountain; the river, its channel in the soil; the animal, its bones in the stratum; the fern and leaf, their modest epitaph in the coal. The falling drop makes its sculpture in the sand or the

stone. Not a foot steps into the snow or along the ground, but prints in characters more or less lasting, a map of its march. Every act of man inscribes itself in the memories of his fellows and in his own manners and face."

References

Anthony, C. P. , & Thebodeau, G. A. Textbook of Anatomy and Physiology. St. Louis: C V Mosby, 1979

Ardell, Donald. High Level Wellness. Berkeley Ten Speed Press, 1977

Briggs, D. C. Celebrate Your Self. Doubleday, New York: 1977

Brunner, L. S. , & Suddarth, D. S. Textbook of Medical - Surgical Nursing. J B Lippincott, New York: 1975

Carson, Richard D. . Taming Your Gremlin. Harper Row, New York: 1983

Cousins, Norman. Anatomy of an Illness. Bantam Books, New York: 1979

Cousins, Norman. Head First. Penquin Books, New York 1990

Frankl, Viktor. Man's Search For Meaning. Simon & Schuster, New York: 1963

Kubler-Ross, Elisabeth. On Death and Dying. New York: Macmillan, 1969

Nursing 79 Books Horsham, PA. Coping With Neurologic Problems Proficiently. Intermed Communications, 1979

Ornstein, Robert, & Sobel, David. The Healing Brain. Simon & Schuster, New York: 1987

Pearsall, Paul. Super Immunity. McGraw Hill, New York: 1987

Siegal, Bernie S. . Love, Medicine and Miracles. Harper & Row, New York: 1986

Smith, Anthony. The Body. Walker & C0. , New York 1968

Springhouse Press. Nurses Clinical Library. Springhouse Corp. , 1984

Thoreau, Henry David. Walden and Civil Disobedience. Airmont Publishing, New York: 1965

Tubesing, Donald, & Tubesing, N. L. The Caring Question. Augsburg Publishing House, Minneapolis: 1983

Vanauken, Sheldon. A Severe Mercy. Bantam, New York: 1977

GLOSSARY

Acetone	fluid having a fruity smell, used as a solvent.
Adrenalin	hormone secreted by the adrenal glands, acts on the smooth muscles and raises blood pressure.
Alveolar	pertaining to the alveoli.
Alveoli	the small sac-like structures in the lungs that allow for oxygen and carbon dioxide exchange.
Aneurysm	a sac, filled with blood, that forms on the wall of a vein or artery.
Anti-pyretic	something that is used to lower body temperature.
Aorta	the large artery that leaves the left side of the heart.

Arachnoid	the middle layer of the meninges, which covers the brain.
Atherosclerosis	narrowing of the arteries caused by accumulation of fatty plaques.
Atria	the upper chambers of the heart.
Atrium	one upper chamber of the heart.
Biot's	a type of breathing rate characterized by rapid breathing followed by no breathing.
Bronchioles	the smaller branches of the tube system in the lungs.
Bronchitis	an inflammation of the bronchus.
Bronchus	the large tube-like structure that carries air from the neck into the lungs.
Broncho-spasm	a closing of the bronchus causing breathing difficulty.
Cardiomyopathy	a disease of the heart muscle of unknown cause.
Cardiovascular	pertaining to the heart and blood vessels.
Cerebellum	small lobe of the brain sitting below the cerebrum and concerned with coordinating movement.
Cerebrum	in human, the largest part of the brain, extends from the front of the skull to the back of the head. Concerned with all rational

	activity as well as feeling and moving specific body parts.
Cheyne-stokes	irregular breathing rate characterized by increasing rate and depth of breathing to a point, then decreasing rate and depth until there in a pause in breathing and the cycle repeats.
Chordotomy	surgical severing of certain tracts of the spinal cord to relieve severe pain.
Clysis	administration of fluid into the skin.
Colitis	an inflammation of the colon.
Convolution	the fold, twist and coil of parts of the brain.
COPD	chronic obstructive pulmonary disease.
CVA	cerebral, vascular accident or stroke.
Dehydrated	insufficient fluid in the tissues of the body.
Detoxify	removal of toxins.
Dialysis	removal of toxins from the body by artificial means when the kidneys are not able to do this adequately.

Diverticulosis	small sac formations in the intestines.
Duodenum	the first part of the small intestines.
Dystrophy	a degeneration, defect or abnormal development.
Edema	swelling due to excessive collection of fluid.
Emboli	undissolved matter floating in the blood vessels.
Embolism	the blockage of a vessel from an embolus.
Embolus	a single emboli.
Emphysema	chronic lung disease characterized by enlarged air sacs.
Endocarditis	an inflammation of the lining of the heart.
Endocardium	the lining of the heart.
Exacerbation	an increase in the severity of a disease.
Expiration	the breathing out of air.
Fibrillation	an uncoordinated twitching of muscles usually refers to an action of the heart muscle.
Fibrosis	an enlarging of connective tissue.
Gastric	pertaining to the stomach.

Gland	a cell, tissue or organ that produces secretions.
Hydrochloric acid	a sharp swelling, corrosive acid found in the stomach to aid digestion.
Hypothalamus	gray matter at the base of the brain. It regulates functions like water balance, temperature and sleep.
Insulin	a hormone secreted by the pancreas. It is needed to metabolize carbohydrates.
Intravenous	within a vein.
Ischemia	decrease in blood supply due to an obstruction or constriction of the vessel.
Larynx	the area, between the back of the tongue and the trachea, which contains the voice box.
Meninges	the covering of the brain and spinal cord.
Meningitis	an inflammation of the covering of the brain and/or spinal cord.
Metabolism	the breaking down of foodstuff into simple products to be used for energy and cell building.
Metastasize	a transfer of a disease from the original site to another part of the body.

Mottling	a discoloration without a distinct pattern.
Mucus	a thick, sticky secretion.
Myocardial	pertaining to the muscle of the heart.
Myocardium	the muscle tissue of the heart.
Neurologic	pertaining to the nervous system.
Neuromuscular	pertaining to the nerves and the muscles.
Node	a small round organ.
Occuled	stopped up, closed off.
Oxygenate	to saturate a substance with oxygen.
Pacemaker	any object that influences the rate of a process of reaction.
Parasympathic	pertaining to the brain concerned with the autonomic nervous system.
Pericardium	the closed sac that holds the heart.
Peristalsis	a progressive wave of contraction seen in the intestines.
Peritonitis	an inflammation of the lining of the abdominal cavity.
Pharynx	the tube that leads from the back of the nose and mouth to the larynx.

Psychoneuroimmunology	the science that studies the relationship among the emotions, the brain and the immune system.
Pulmonary	pertaining to or affecting the lungs.
Pylorus	the circular opening between the stomach and the small intestines.
Sclerosis	hardening of a part due to overgrowth of fibrous tissue.
Thrombus	a clot of blood formed within the heart or blood vessels.
TIA	(transicent ischemia attack) a temporary interruption of blood flow usually due to spasm of a vessel.
Trachea	the tube that extends from the larynx to the bronchi.
Tubules	a small tube.
Turgor	the normal texture of the skin.
Ulcerative	characterized by an interruption of the normal tissue.
Ureters	the tubes leading from the kidneys to the bladder.
Urethra	the tube leading from the bladder to outside the body. In the female it is one and a half inches long. In the males it is 8 to 9 inches long.

Urinary	pertaining to urine.
Vena	vein.
Ventricle	the lower chambers of the heart.
Ventricular	pertaining to the ventricle.

www.ingramcontent.com/pod-product-compliance
Lightning Source LLC
Chambersburg PA
CBHW030014190526
45157CB00016B/2722